HELP YOURSELF!

For over three-quarters of a century the Bircher-
Benner Clinic of Zurich, Switzerland has been the
center of nutritional treatment of disease. Its staff
of physicians and specialists has developed an
internationally acclaimed program of meal plan-
ning, treatment and physical fitness that is outlined
in this series of outstanding health guides.

The *Plan for High Blood Pressure Problems* contains everything you need to know about the silent
killers that have become a national health disaster:
arteriosclerosis and high blood pressure diseases.
Contrary to popular belief, they are not merely
diseases of the aging. Recent medical evidence
has proven that the pattern for arteriosclerosis
can begin in infancy and be well advanced in the
earliest years of life, particularly among teenage
males.

The information in this book may save your life.
No family should be without it.

ABOUT THE
BIRCHER-BENNER CLINIC

In the nineteenth century, Dr. M. Bircher-Benner established a kind of clinic that had never existed before: a clinic that would take into account the whole man, body and soul, not only the patient's disease; a clinic that would use an intelligent patient as a co-worker in a total therapeutic effort; a clinic that would use the total knowledge of modern medicine to support the "internal physician"—the autonomous healing forces and healing system of the body—and in every case make the healing effects of dietetic therapy and one's life-style the basis of a total health plan; a clinic that, in addition to eliminating immediate ailments, would bring about a new, tougher, more satisfying and creative health of body and soul for the patient.

The private clinic founded in 1897 by Dr. Bircher-Benner is still operated today for that purpose.

Bircher-Benner Nutrition Plan for High Blood Pressure Problems

A Comprehensive Guide With Suggestions for Diet Menus and Recipes

Translated by Kenneth C. Taylor

By the staff of the Bircher-Benner Clinic:

Medical/Dietetic Section:
D. Liechti-v. Brasch, M.D.,
P. F. Boesch, M.D.,
S. Grieder-Dopheide, M.D.

Physiological/Chemical Section:
Alfred Kunz-Bircher, Ph.D.

Menus and Recipes:
Ruth Kunz-Bircher, M.D.
(head of the Bircher-Benner Clinic)

Edited by Ralph Bircher, M.D.

PYRAMID PUBLICATIONS 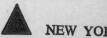 NEW YORK

BIRCHER-BENNER NUTRITION PLAN FOR
HIGH BLOOD PRESSURE PROBLEMS
A PYRAMID BOOK

Originally published in German under the title BIRCHER-BENNER-
HANDBUCH FUR ARTERIOSKLEROSE-UND BLUTHOCHDRUCKKRANKE

Copyright © 1973 by Nash Publishing

Pyramid edition published January 1977

ISBN: 0-515-04228-5

Library of Congress Catalog Card Number: 72-81864

Printed in the United States of America

_____

Pyramid Books are published by Pyramid Publications (Harcourt Brace
Jovanovich). Its trademarks, consisting of the word "Pyramid" and the
portrayal of a pyramid, are registered in the United States Patent Office.

Pyramid Publications (Harcourt Brace Jovanovich).
757 Third Avenue, New York, N.Y. 10017

Contents

I. Introduction

Of all illnesses, few in our time are so widespread, few remove as many people prematurely from work and from life, and few bring so much grief and sorrow to the lives of innumerable families as does the group of high blood pressure ailments and arteriosclerosis. Yet, only relatively few people thus afflicted obtain medical treatment, all too often after the disease has progressed so far that full recovery is hardly ever possible. For it is a characteristic of these diseases to progress unobserved for decades without producing complaints or noticeable symptoms. This is the so-called iceberg phenomenon, only one-tenth of which emerges from the sea, while nine-tenths are submerged and invisible. In arteriosclerosis and hypertension, only a twentieth of the whole is open to view; the remaining 19/20 remain imperceptible, the disorder, still in its symptom-free phase, is hidden, but built in (D. M. Spain, Columbia University). Health is only an illusion while, in reality, more or less serious pathological disorders exist, still masked, often by very efficient systems the organism is endowed with in order to compensate for, regulate, or bypass the disorder.

The results of autopsies performed on 300 *young* American soldiers (abundant rations, rich in animal fats and proteins; heavy smokers), killed during the Korean war, are of great significance here. Not just a few, but more than three quarters (77.3%) of them were found to have "very obvious sclerosis of the coronary vessels of the heart, with fibrotic thickening of large atheromatous spots and

7

complete occlusion of one or more coronary vessels"—in short, a well-developed, even if concealed, early stage of arteriosclerosis—and that, in spite of an average age of only 22.1 years! At this age, it can be another 20-25 years before serious disturbances from vessel degeneration require medical intervention. Among the native soldiers of the South Korean army (short rations with little animal protein and fat) conditions such as those found in the Americans were almost entirely lacking.

Similarly relevant are the results of the Peckham investigations on 2000 healthy families (40% children!). An especially impressive example was that of a 21-year-old sports enthusiast, training for a title in boxing, and such a picture of health and fitness that no one, least of all himself, would have thought he was ailing. But examination showed a blood pressure of 230 (instead of 120) mm Hg and seriously endangered kidneys! Ninety percent of the healthy individuals examined by Peckham showed more or less serious health problems of various types.

Arteriosclerosis and high blood pressure have long been considered inevitable diseases of old age; but this view has been renounced since it is no longer substantiated by the facts. The number of cases far exceeds the shift in superannuation of the population. Mortality from this group of diseases increased in Switzerland from 30% before World War II to 40% in 1954 and today in the USA comprises already 55% of insurance cases. In Great Britain in only 4 years (1947-1951) it rose 57% from 38,000 to 58,000. The number of patients stricken with heart attacks has increased 5-fold in 20 years as Professor Hochrein (Ludwigshafen) reported, based on his clinical material. Autopsy of a cross section of war-dead in World War I (American Army 1917) which corresponded to the Korean investigation of 1951 in every respect, revealed that 45% of the young soldiers examined at that time had the described degenerative changes of the vascular system, in 1951, 77.3%. According to reports of the Louisiana Faculty of Medicine in April 1956, such degenerative changes can now even be confirmed in children. Not long ago a 2-day-old infant died in a children's hospital of coronary sclerosis and cardiac infarction.

A large American study (W. Dock) shows that an elevated cholesterol level, clogging and degeneration of vessels occur very early in young American males, increasing rapidly from about the eleventh year of age to a maximum at 19 years. "At 30 years the average male has hardening of the coronary arteries, which is 65% as serious as the condition to which men succumb at age 50; and at 50 years of age the average approaches (in degree of seriousness) 82% of the fatal infiltration of the intima." Another study (University of New Orleans) on nearly 12,000 very healthy, trouble-free young men (20-49 years old) found, on the basis of routine examinations, that 41.5% had serious cardiac, circulatory and renal disorders of which the individual was unaware. On the other hand, many investigations have established that in several continents there are scattered populations which remain free from hypertension and arteriosclerosis, until old age, even in the hidden, built-in phases of these ailments. Their nutritional habits were investigated, and diets derived therefrom that efficiently cure and prevent these diseases (e.g., the "Oriental Diet," Framingham, Ohio). In the Bircher-Banner medical center, since its foundation in 1897, both worldwide research and clinical experience in this field have been accumulated and integrated, so that more than the usual treatment can be applied. In many cases, full recovery is attained when the patient is given treatment early enough, often in cases where success seemed out of reach. At the least, the progress of the disease is halted. The best chances for full recovery and lifelong good health exist, of course, when the treatment can be applied in the "underground" phase, or when the disease has just begun to emerge. Incidentally, the patient can, by this treatment, overcome not only the particular disease, but may enjoy a general boost of his life force and stamina. Still, the changeover according to the advice contained in this book is rewarding even to the patient in advanced phases, by improving his condition and spurring a fresh blossoming of his mental and physical capacities.

All these findings point to several important considerations. First, that these diseases have a very long and imperceptible progress in the preliminary stage. Secondly, that the human organism must have an almost inexhaustible capacity to compensate for these disturbances and damages, so that the life and functioning of the individual appears unimpaired for a long time. Quietly producing and diligently adjusting, year after year, the body assumes the burden of increasing difficulties and renders them unnoticeable to us, so long as the system functions somehow. The mind is hardly capable of understanding these changes, and we are indebted to the Creator for giving us an organism the extent of whose capabilities few among us can comprehend.

However, a great tragedy is inherent in the fact of the body's unprecedented compensatory mechanisms. The instant that the disease finally becomes a visible threat and a physician is needed, it may often be too late for complete recovery. Even if the worst can be prevented, damage and debilitation may occur which may always partially persist. In this case, the patient must learn to live with his disease. He should be happy to have come out alive and to know how he can best utilize his remaining strength and potentialities for the future. Medical remedies offer a few short-term possibilities in preventing a crisis; sometimes a skillful surgeon can bring relief at the cost of crippling. But the only way in which a real recovery can be affected is by means of, what Dr. Bircher-Benner has called, "regulation therapy". This involves a new way of life which follows life's own rules of order and advances the vital regulative powers of body, mind and soul. This is possible through the skillful cooperation of physician and patient in the service of life's own powers of self-recovery. A greater, superhuman power and wisdom must intercede in our behalf, because, as Dr. Bircher-Benner writes, "There is a noble and powerful wisdom which functions within man himself but is concealed to our eyes. It alone can maintain and reestablish health."

First of all, the physician must, of course, thoroughly and precisely examine the situation and prevent any danger, in order to gain time. He will establish a treatment plan which must be geared to the patient's characteristics and reactions, and he will clarify its significance for the patient. All in all, this is not a mean, but rather a very demanding task which requires maturity, knowledge and ability.

The patient, for his part, must learn the situation as it is. He must know that, now, he no longer has "the gift of plenty"; the reserves have become limited, sometimes very limited, and the way has become narrow. He must now become knowledgeable about his organism and must learn to budget his life.

He must also know that by this method he will have prospects for enjoyment, which no other method can even approach. To what extent recovery is possible in individual cases and the extent to which the circulatory system will regain its former capabilities remain to be determined. This depends upon several conditions, not the least of which are attitude and insight of the patient himself; despite "built-in weaknesses" which cannot be entirely removed, he will still be able to lead a long, productive and, perhaps, an especially worthwhile life, if he learns to live *with* his organism instead of *against* it. The following information serves this purpose.

How to face environmental pollution: Like a dark cloud, the menace of air, water, soil, and food pollution hovers over us, but the individual and his family are not nearly so helpless in the face of this threat as many believe. Of course, it will take a long time for industry and the state to restore, or even stabilize the environment, to make it more bearable and, even, danger-free—and the financial burden will be heavy. In the meantime, however, each one of us can do a lot to enhance his organism's resistance by helping his body's natural capacity for decontamination. Unwittingly, most of us abuse and heavily overtax the systems the organism is endowed with to fight contamination. For those who understand this, and act accordingly, the environmental threat loses much of its weight. This book will help you to do so. For example, remember that animal foods, especially meat and fish, are much more contaminated than vegetable foods, especially by systemic ("in-built") substances and, tragically, contaminated, since the transition to industrial meat and egg production, by antiobiotics, hormones, arsenicals, lead, mercury, fattening chemicals, tranquillizers, tenderizers, chemical aromatic substances, carcinogens, thyreostatics, preservatives, and pesticides. Whoever can, should, of course, try to provide himself and his family with unpolluted foods, organically grown by himself, on his own ground—but not everyone can, like the Scott Nearings, leave the city behind to live in the country. But he can, and should, at least do what this book recommends to decontaminate his body and improve its stamina. Much more can be accomplished than most people imagine is possible.

All of the above points to the necessity of providing the patient with a thorough, yet brief and comprehensible manual, which during treatment will facilitate work with the physician and, afterwards, will permit further improvement. This manual will guide him with respect to the conditions for his health, the suitability of his food, the pursuit of his diet and other practical measures which can also be carried out at home. The diet must continue to be entirely satisfying, even when it complies with the requirements of the altered situation, and it must afford a maximum of restorative capability. Such a manual should complement the physician's orders and advise the patient how to deal with his organism, to prevent relapses and to continue to strengthen his health. It contains many objectives which are very important for his future, and he will not regret giving his complete attention to the following exposition.

ARTERIOSCLEROSIS

In recent years, specialists have made significant progress in elucidating how the alterations occur which lead to arteriosclerosis, so that, today, we have some insight into what is happening. The disease begins with degeneration of the inner walls of the blood vessels of the entire vascular system. The degenerating walls appear to attract the fatty substance, cholesterol, from the blood which, together with albumin, is deposited so that the vessel walls thicken, the functional diameter is reduced and blood flow is obstructed. At the same time, they lose their original flexibility, and this can progress to the point where the organism must take precautionary means in order to prevent catastrophes from torn blood vessels: Calcium is deposited to strengthen the vessel walls.

The nature of the fatty deposits on the inner walls of the vessels has been investigated, and it was found that they consist primarily of cholesterol. It was also found that their formation is doubtlessly enhanced by an excess of cholesterol in the blood (plasma cholesterol). A high cholesterol level always implies danger of arteriosclerosis.

What factors are responsible for an elevated plasma cholesterol level? Cholesterol is an indispensable substance in the machinery of the body, since it is the precursor in the formation of bile acids, adrenal hormones, sex hormones and the antirachitic Vitamin D_3. It is also an indispensable component of every body cell. The body by itself is normally capable of satisfying its cholesterol requirement by synthesis in the liver and in the intestinal mucosa, and it also has at its disposal techniques for catabolism and excretion of cholesterol in the feces. A central regulatory mechanism maintains equilibrium between the synthesis and catabolism of cholesterol and assures that plasma cholesterol remains at correct physiological levels. If absorption is interfered with for any reason, or if cholesterol is ingested, then less is formed in the body, and vice versa.

Cholesterol can be obtained from (animal) food. It has been shown that the body's own production of cholesterol in the liver and intestinal wall is reduced or stops entirely as cholesterol is administered. Recent investigations (Blankenhorn, University of California) showed that the cholesterol deposited on the inner walls of vessels is most probably entirely derived from administered animal foods.

We have seen that the plasma cholesterol level is regulated by the body; however, it seems that this regulation is limited. In man it is only of limited efficiency, otherwise it would not fail so early in the majority of civilized men. It has been shown that in meat-eating animals, e.g., in rats, it is much more efficient than in man, since it has not been possible to raise cholesterol levels in these animals with cholesterol-rich feed. On the other hand, in apes, rabbits and other vegetarians, cholesterol levels can be raised as in man. These circumstances led several investigators to postulate that man's disposition for arteriosclerosis is further evidence that man was originally a fruit eater, as his teeth also show, although he has a unique capacity for adaptation. But even the greatest adaptive capabilities must not be continually overworked. For this reason the prevention and cure of arteriosclerosis require that the vital conditions for natural elimination be approximated, in order that the regulatory mechanisms not be overburdened; i.e., in this case that the intake of animal foods be diminished.

Cholesterol only occurs in animal foods, primarily in fats, and in the following amounts (according to Professor Halden):

milligrams	per 100 g
12	milk
140	cheese
240	butter
120-280	meat
480	eggs
670	goose liver (fattened)
2360	brain

Thus, whoever avoids animal foods also avoids ingestion of cholesterol. Some have even gone so far, for the sake of preventing and curing arteriosclerosis, to entirely forbid or avoid all animal fats if not all animal foods. This is unnecessary and makes the diet unnecessarily difficult. As we have already indicated above, the plasma cholesterol level can be rapidly lowered to normal even when some animal fats and foods containing cholesterol are consumed in moderation. A too strict procedure will, in many cases, lead to danger.

More important than the amount of the cholesterol

supply is the nature of the dietary cholesterol, its *quality*. The liver of a highly fattened goose provides 670 mg cholesterol in 100 gm while the liver of a healthy goose provides only 70 mg; moreover, that 670 mg consists, for the most part, of beta-lipoproteins and *only the beta-lipoproteins tend toward deposition on the arterial walls*, while the alpha-lipoproteins have every quality which benefits the human body. There is a striking difference in the ratio of alpha-to-beta. In the rat it amounts to 70/30, in man almost the reverse, 28/72, at least in young, healthy individuals in whom cholesterol regulation still functions. However, there are other young people who have ratios of 9/91 in favor of the poorly tolerated beta-lipoproteins.

Until recently, the notion prevailed that the *fat content* of food was the major factor responsible for the occurrence of arteriosclerosis, irrespective of whether it is animal or vegetable fat. Today we know that it is *animal fat* which is responsible and that *vegetable fat can even contribute to a reduction in cholesterol levels if it is rich in polyunsaturated fatty acids.*

Above all, a person endangered by arteriosclerosis should know that the *polyunsaturated fatty acids and vitamin E can be preventative and therapeutic for this disease.* He should also know that the spread of this ailment in recent times is intimately associated with the fact—as pointed out by Professor Sinclair, a nutrition physiologist of Oxford University—that the nutrition of affluent civilized peoples continues to become not only richer in quantity and in animal fat, but also richer in saturated, chemically produced and unnatural fatty acids and poorer in the essential fatty acids (EFA). The hard fats and refined oils can even act as antivitamins. It requires about 2 g of polyunsaturated fatty acids to undo the damage caused by 1 g of saturated fatty acid. Vitamin E and polyunsaturated fatty acids are most abundant in whole wheat, whole soya, germinated grains, wheat-germ oil, nuts and natural oils from linseed and sunflower kernels and sesame. The fat ration of the diet must be carefully chosen from these fats and fatty agents. It is not sufficient to merely add a large quantity of polyunsaturated fatty acids to one's normal diet or to improve an excessively rich fat ration with fatty acids of this type. Although this will reduce the cholesterol content by 23% within 5 months (Indiana experiment), it will lead to fatty degeneration of the liver, and when, because of this, the diet must be stopped the patient will be worse off than before.

The *lecithins* are also *substances which protect against arteriosclerosis*. These are highly valuable fats containing phosphate, which, in limited amounts, fulfill several important functions in the organism. The more lecithin is supplied in the diet, the less harmful becomes the cholesterol intake, and the less the chance of regulatory mechanisms failing. Lecithin is found mainly in green leaves, whole wheat, soya, nuts and milk, but not in butter, since almost the entire lecithin content of milk goes to *buttermilk*.

Milk and buttermilk are valuable to those ailing from arteriosclerosis, due to their high content of the amino acid, *methionine,* which counteracts excess cholesterol. It is, therefore, advisable not to exclude the low-fat dairy products from the diet of those endangered with arteriosclerosis.

The importance of proteins: Protein is a factor that also has to be considered in the formation of arteriosclerosis. Excessive protein intake, especially of animal protein, and most of all of meat protein, decisively contributes to the genesis of athermatosis. This was discovered in the U.S. at the end of the fifties and in the newer amyloidosis research. Amyloidosis—"the most important and perhaps decisive cause of health decline in aging"—appears to be the formation of deteriorated proteins and fats. The sebacious and greasy deposits, called amyloid, pervading the body, contain certain amino acids in excess. Amino acids are contained in veal, for instance, 4½ times more than in walnuts, although the protein percentage is quite similar insofar as tyrosin is concerned, and even 5½ times more as concerns tryptophan. Excess protein—the body needs not more than 50 to 60 grams per day for full health—is not used for body substance replacement but for energy production, and must be burned rapidly. Therefore, the excess acts in a way similar to pressing the gas lever in a motor car. It produces a hypermetabolizing effect which is felt as stimulation, but becomes a stress factor when habitually repeated. Incidentally, the organism is charged with toxic breaking-down substances from protein decay which cannot be eliminated rapidly enough. Thus they are supposedly contributing to amyloid formation.

Fortunately the organism is endowed with a defense system against amyloidosis, but this regulator soon breaks down if it is claimed heavily for long periods of time, which is almost generally the case with nutritional habits as they exist in today's affluent societies. It breaks down, especially, when further toxic substances from digestive putrefaction add their influence—which also stems mainly from an excessive intake of animal proteins and lack of vegetable roughage. An autoimmune reaction is then ensured in the intercellular tissues (mesenchyme) which enhances the amyloidose. The causal connection between animal protein and amyloidose is easily demonstrated in experiments with animals.

The importance of carbohydrates: A number of research workers hold that carbohydrates also play a major role in originating arteriosclerosis, and many results appear to support this view insofar as the carbohydrates in question are white sugar, and other refined carbohydrates as consumed in great excess in these days. Sugar, especially, in refined and concentrated form deranges the functioning of the organism, diverts vitamins and deranges fat and protein metabolism so that these nutrients cannot be efficiently used. We hold, that one may insist not too much on reducing, or even avoiding, habitual intake of refined carbohydrates to adopt instead wholegrain cereals and natural sources of sweetness, like fruits, if these diseases are to be cured and prevented. All depends on a harmonious and well-balanced whole metabolism and food intake. Special caution to be taken against refined carbohydrates is to be recommended to that part of the population which by constitution tends towards insulinism.

Accelerated growth: More than twenty years ago, nutritional science decided that nature had "flunked its exams" by providing far too little protein for mother's milk. Breastfeeding was not advised and artificial baby food flooded the market, containing threefold percentage of protein (and too much salt and sugar). In the meantime, the drawbacks of this error became evident. Babies already had excess amounts of such amino acids as lead to amyloidosis, and they were trained from birth in the wrong direction, i.e., towards poor protein economy, and later protein craving, enhanced by overfeeding with refined carbohydrates. Thus they got sick earlier. It is worthwhile, then, to begin with arteriosclerosis prevention in the infant stage, if not during pregnancy.

A further drawback was even more accelerated growth during childhood, causing premature puberty and retarding mental maturity, with all the educational problems which ensue. The increase of red globules, which had been a main argument in favor of the meat-enriched baby foods, has proved to be a main cause of the tendency towards arteriosclerosis—which is, the greater number of red globules. Autopsies at Columbia University showed that 10% of the babies and toddlers already had heart disorders. "The evidence is accumulating, that degenerative diseases commence earlier." Therefore, it is wise to train children in protein economy and to preserve them from insulinism, being very careful with sweets and refined carbohydrates. This book helps to do so, showing how to satisfy their desire for sweetness with fresh fruits, and how to offer them appetizing roughage of all kinds, nuts, and protein combinations of highest biological value as potatoes with milk, whole grains with leafy vegetables, pulses with corn, for "mixtures of two proteins always have a higher value than each of its components." Thus, the revolutionary discoveries that arose from the researches carried out at the Max Planck Institute for Nutritional Physiology were made public.

Vitamin B, *nicotine acid amide* (vitamin PP, Niacin, anti-pellagra factor) has a marked influence in reducing cholesterol. One difficulty that normally occurs in combatting pellagra with this vitamin arises not from insufficient supply but rather from interference with its utilization, as may occur in albumin-rich diets, alcoholism, high sugar intake and in diarrhea. With administration of nicotinic acid amide, the cholesterol level can be reduced within 6 weeks from 290 to 232 mg, i.e., about 20%.

Satiation of the organism with *vitamin* C can considerably reduce cholesterol levels. This is most readily achieved through suitable fresh fruit juices and vegetable juices.

Considerable reduction in cholesterol levels can also be achieved by a diet rich in *alkaline mineral substances* such as potassium and silicon, and *low in acidic mineral substances,* such as sodium and calcium. Degeneration of the arterial walls can be measured by its silicon content. This diet proposed in this handbook is especially rich in alkalis.

Apples are especially useful in the battle against arteriosclerosis. The *pectin* content of 2 apples (15 g) is able to reduce cholesterol levels by 10 mg (Ancel Keys).

The trace element *magnesium* (in nuts) is also very useful in this respect. It lowers cholesterol by mobilizing organelles in living cells against excess acidity in the tissues and towards phosphate absorption in the body.

Recent experimental results clearly demonstrate that (given the same circumstances) *animal protein*—meat, eggs, cheese—raises cholesterol levels while *vegetable protein*—nuts, grain, vegetables, legumes, soya—lowers cholesterol levels and cures the arterial degeneration.

Besides the intake of animal fat and high-cholesterol foods there is a series of other influences which contribute to damage of the arterial walls and lead to disease. These include strongly *spiced foods,* daily consumption of *stimulants and intoxicants, addiction to medication, the carbon monoxide effect of smoking, breathing polluted air, the continuous production of toxins by impacted teeth and other hidden infections in the body, lack of exercise and sleep, a hectic, anxious and unfulfilled life, as well as hereditary predisposition.* All of these work together and must be kept in mind. Last but not least: excess food. Average food consumption is much higher than the actual requirement.

Medical experience shows that the arteriosclerotic is usually a person who "can stand everything," who tolerates fatty foods and who indulges heartily at meals. Nothing prevents him from indulging in the usual habits of eating, drinking, smoking and enjoyment with many rich foods, meats, sweets and canned foods. However, there are also persons who prefer to eat more simply, but who eat all sorts of snacks at all times.

Craving for food and overweight usually accompany excess consumption of stimulants, alcoholic beverages, sweets, abuse of laxatives, analgesics and narcotics, a degenerating intestinal flora and a sluggish and disturbed digestion, liver dysfunction, irritability and internal unrest. Some people seem unable to get away from city routines; for instance, to walk in the country or even a park; they are easily depressed by troubles and disappointments and are prone to face life with distrust. To help such patients requires a large measure of patience, skill and confidence on the part of the physician, the nurse and the relatives.

HIGH BLOOD PRESSURE DISEASE

An increase in blood pressure and general vascular tension is associated with the development of arteriosclerotic changes in the circulatory system. This can be readily understood from the preceding discussion. However, the blood pressure elevation may be moderate, remaining within the "normal" range. This is illustrated by the Eskimo hunters of eastern Greenland. Arteriosclerosis begins very early in these people and achieves dangerously high degrees of arterial change by the third decade of their lives (the food of these Eskimos is nevertheless meager and mostly uncooked, but very rich in animal protein and fat). Despite this their blood pressure is rarely higher than what is considered "normal" for Western civilizations (because it corresponds to the middle-age average and remains without external symptoms of disease). If these Eskimos are compared with other primitive peoples who live, not by hunting, but rather from farming, there is a significant difference in blood pressure. It appears, that there is evidently a different, lower, norm which does not increase with age. This is the norm which we consider to be *real*, whereas the higher norm which is valid professionally is the one for "civilized" peoples. The exact level of the *real* norm for blood pressure and cholesterol must still be determined. The people of Hunza (Tibet) may still provide this opportunity.

On the other hand, a vegetarian monastic order or an African tribe who eat poor diets, low in protein and fat, were found to have hardly any arteriosclerotic degeneration nor elevated blood cholesterol levels; but they did have higher blood pressure, on the average, due to abundant salt intake.

The people of eastern Greenland lead an "uncivilized" life in a very hostile environment which makes severe demands on the adaptability of the human organism. Their food is in a natural state, i.e., uuprocessed. But it consists mainly of fat meat from wild, rather than domesticated animals. Had they been eating meat from fattened domesticated animals, these Eskimos would long since have become extinct. Even so, their diet is evidently inappropriate for the human constitution. Otherwise, they would not have degenerative symptoms at such an early age.

Blood pressure rises as a *life maintaining necessity* for the organism. If it did not rise, the blood supply to the organs would be insufficient. In healthy people blood pressure is maintained at normal levels by central regulation. After each deviation this regulatory mechanism provides for the rapid and complete return to normal. There arise repeated demand situations in life which require an intense increase in functional capacity of the blood; this is accompanied by a temporary elevation of blood pressure. The vital organs must be supplied with more blood. But this cannot last forever and the norm must be re-established, otherwise, recovery would be impaired and the heart and circulation would be "worn out." Particularly in sleep, blood pressure is lowered to a minimum level.

But the regulation of blood pressure in man, like that of the cholesterol level, appears to be only *relatively* effective, as is evident from the alarming problem of blood pressure diseases in our time.

However, chronically elevated blood pressure can also occur as a side effect of various organic diseases. This must first be confirmed by a physician. Organic diseases are the cause in only 5% of cases. Thus, in 95% of cases an *actual blood pressure disease* is involved. For these there is no other known basis than impaired regulation.

Even when no specific organ disease is involved (e.g., a kidney ailment), the kidneys do play a role in the disease. Blood must always pass through the kidneys, as in a filter, to be cleansed of toxic substances. If this filter is continuously overburdened, more adrenalin is secreted into the blood. This hormone accelerates blood flow and increases blood pressure to prepare the body for increased activity. This also occurs in anger, fright and vexation and with every mental and physical stress.

With continuous overloading of the kidneys, blood pressure rises to force filtration. Most people are unaware that excess intake of protein in the form of protein-rich foods (meats, cheese, eggs) severely burdens the kidneys and produces an elevation in blood pressure. Abundant consumption of meat intensifies this effect due to irritative action of substances which can be extracted from meat juices and often also from roasted meats. The liver is then overburdened by an abundance of protein. This amounts to, at least, 30%.

An additional cause for recurring increases in blood pressure is pus-producing foci in the teeth or tonsils, for example. These can sometimes cause a marked elevation of blood pressure in quite young people. Furthermore, the continuous effects of carbon monoxide in smokers increases vascular constriction, as does the action of metabolic toxins which arise from protein-rich diets or altered intestinal flora and which, in time, gain access to the blood.

Experience shows that a diet in which meat dishes play a major role induces more food intake and heavier use of seasoning and salt; that it, moreover, damages the bacterial flora of the intestine, especially when the diet is low in fresh foods. Excessive food and salt intake is a burden which can produce elevation in blood pressure.

Thus, it is understandable that the usual meat and animal protein diet frequently promotes blood pressure disease. Research supports this, such as has been done with monks from various orders, or Chinese or blacks who have settled in the USA after leaving their homelands and have acquired a new way of life; or observations on athletes who eat much meat, or the well-known personal experiment of Dr. Bienstock; but the clearest proof was provided by Mayer and Gudzeit in an extensive investigation carried out in 1944 in Breslau. They compared the diet and blood pressure of 2500 butchers who, at that time, despite five years of strict rationing, were still able to obtain abundant meat, with an equal number of citizens who could obtain only 1/4 to 1/12 as much animal protein. This investigation was carried out with great care and, due to the unusual circumstances and precautions, allowed *"the compelling conclusion that blood pressure rises in proportion to the intake of animal protein."*

In a few cases there may be another primary cause for the rise in blood pressure: *Disturbed emotional balance.* When a person in no longer able to achieve a meaningful relationship with his environment in the rush of daily life; or when his life is filled with tension or pent-up anger; when he can no longer master his goals and tasks; when he suffers set-backs and disappointments and must endure counter pressure and emotional tension; when all this is constantly repeated, then blood pressure can become fixed at an abnormally high level. This may occur even without any other contributing cause, and, at first, may be only a temporary elevation which later becomes permanent. These irritations always induce the secretion of adrenalin into the blood and similarly reinforce the effects discussed above.

In addition, congenital and acquired conditions naturally work together in all of this. Thus, increases in blood pressure may occur late and weakly in some individuals, earlier and more severely in others and, in still others, an abnormal fall in blood pressure may occur. The latter has been observed more frequently in recent times; regulatory mechanisms are worn out.

We maintain, nevertheless, that dietary habits are the main underlying factor in the disease and thus, as a rule, are of concern for effective prevention and treatment.

When the normal diet is such that it prevent arteriosclerosis and high blood pressure, then anxiety and mental problems are of little or no effect. ("Presidential Address," *Journal of the American Medical Association*.)

Chronic high blood pressure constricts the fine blood vessels like a slow, perfidious setscrew, so that they become narrower and narrower, and, finally, no longer allow blood to flow through. The blood, however, circulates in a closed system without an overflow valve, and pressure must inevitably rise. If it becomes too high and the elasticity of the vessel walls diminishes, then they must be strengthened. This is, however, not possible without their becoming hardened, and, finally the increased pressure may cause them to rupture somewhere, be it in the brain, the heart, the kidneys or in the eye.

This development can be protracted over years or decades and therefore proceeds without any complaints for a very long time. There are people who, with an exceedingly high blood pressure of 300 mm Hg, do not experience the slightest problem; on the other hand, there are those who, at a moderately elevated blood pressure of 180 mm Hg, feel markedly ill. *The sick person should always be glad that his heart has the strength to overcome the impeding vascular constriction;* but he must bear in mind that this task imposes upon the heart an inevitable and often immense strain.

The human heart so far surpasses all known motors in functional capacity that we can hardly hope to improve on it, even with the most ingenuous machine produced by man. Hochrein describes it vividly: "It works without interruption for 70 or 80 years without care or cleaning, without repair or replacement, day and night. It beats 100,000 times per day, approximately 40 million times in a year and within 70 years supplies the pumping capacity for nearly three billion cardiac pulsations. It pumps 2 gallons of blood per minute and 100 gallons per hour, through a vascular system of about 60,000 miles in length—2-1/2 times the circumference of the earth."* Yet, this is only the resting

---

* In *Doctors Speak to You*, Hans Huber Verlag, Bern.

capacity of the heart. Every stimulus that strikes the body demands from it an increased energy output.

To what extent must this irreplaceable "miracle motor" be misused before it finally breaks down! The number of those suffering from cardiac and circulatory ailments keeps increasing at an even faster rate, far exceeding the displacement in age. Continuous and excessive misuse bears its fruit!

Yet the heart, as Hochrein has pointed out, cannot rest for even a moment. Unlike other muscular organs, which through protective fatigue provide the necessary full recovery, it must continue to pump even in sleep. Its functional capacity is guaranteed by various regulatory mechanisms if relative rest is granted it by maintaining the 24-hour rhythm of day and night. At night, nature's rhythm slows down to a low speed. For eight hours the heart is not confronted with sudden boosts in performance and the demand for work is diminished. All organs work minimally, blood pressure is lower than at any other time, the need for blood flow to the surfaces of all parts of the body is reduced, the coronary vessels are not stressed, all processes are not only reduced in intensity but adjusted to a more economical effort.

Adequate nightly rest is the modest, but essential need of our tireless, continuously active, central, and most vital organ, the heart. This is a basic rule of life of granting this rest and respecting it, we tend to fatally disturb it by going to sleep too late and giving the organism too little relaxation time. All this must be changed in high-blood pressure patients: they must learn to live *with* their hearts, not against them.

GENERAL GUIDELINES
FOR PROMOTING RECOVERY

The *health diet,* outlined here, *therapeutically influences all major conditions simultaneously:* The smallest capillary vessels, arteries, the coronary vessels, the arterioles, the supply of cardiac hormone, the endocrine system, reducing the load of the metabolic and excretory organs and thereby also of the cardiac muscle, the functioning of regulatory mechanisms and the regeneration of interstitial tissue. The results of this diet in arteriosclerosis and high blood pressure disease are most impressive. *As a rule it returns elevated blood cholesterol levels to normal in 4-7 days,* irrespective of whether they are moderately or markedly elevated, *and it normalizes the elevated blood pressure within 15-30 days.*

The diet stresses fresh foods. It uses vegetable oils and fats of highest biological quality (freshly pressed vegetable oil, nut butter, sesame, almond purée, whole soya, nuts, almonds, wheat germ). It contains plenty of vegetables and fruit in the form of fresh juices and salads, which contain substances lowering blood pressure. It uses potato juice, supplies much nicotinic acid and vitamin B_6, vitamin PP, vitamin E and highly unsaturated fatty acids, lecithin and methionine, all of which lower blood pressure and promote the catabolism of cholesterol. It saturates the organisms with citrus which are rich in vitamins C and PP and in the liver-protecting substances, *rutin,* which also contributes to lower blood pressure. It puts great value on herbs, wild greens and fruits and on daily vegetable broth as a mineral-rich, basic, ingredient for all cooked dishes; on sprouted whole grains as an additional ingredient, and above all on a combination of food low in salt and sodium. Prepared thus, it lowers the blood pressure and will be a source of continual enjoyment once one is accustomed to it. It avoids overly concentrated nutrients, and begins, instead, with dishes that are comfortably filling without overloading the organism, so that excess food intake is naturally limited. It does not avoid all animal foods yet still achieves its effects, especially the required reduction in cholesterol intake. It uses, at the most, 20-30 g (1 oz) butter and milk fat, but excludes all denatured fats. It provides animal protein in the form of buttermilk, whey, yogurt and cottage cheese. It emphasizes tasty whole-grain dishes.

This diet, in particular, is low in cooking salt and if necessary, can be prepared entirely without cooking salt and very little sodium. Beyond this, it is particularly rich in potassium and thereby achieves the greatest possible relief for the circulation and interstitial tissues and the greatest possible charge with bio-electric potential. It is generally moderate in fat and protein content and relatively low in animal protein; however it guarantees an ideal supply of both these groups of nutrients, of high quality and highly economical in use. Fat intake amounts to 10-50-90 g (1/2-3 oz) per day depending upon the diet prescribed by the physician. Of course, alcohol, stimulants, tobacco, sweets and fancy pastries must be avoided. It is easier with this diet than with any other. If the subsequent instructions for preparation of foods are carefully followed, the food will be tasty, even completely without salt, and provide so much enjoyment that adherence to the diet even for an unlimited time will be possible.

The internal emergency regulatory changes which were necessary during the disease may continue after the general condition has improved and the heart has recovered and will only gradually make way for healthy regulation. If the diet is stopped during this period and old habits are reassumed, new deteriorations and relapses may occur. Thus, the patient must remember that the unburdening and exercise phase of the therapeutic process, which requires the precise control and instruction of an experienced physician, is followed by a period of regeneration and stabilization which must also run its course.

The health of the *intestine* requires special attention. The physician will provide relief with enemas when necessary. The health diet provides an oxygen-free physiologic intestinal milieu in which a healthy intestinal flora can thrive. When necessary, the diet is supplemented by colonies of functionally capable intestinal bacteria so that food is again used economically, cholesterol catabolism is accelerated, putrefaction and fermentation processes in the intestine cease, and vitamins are abundantly produced by the intestine.

A *regular daily schedule* is essential: Circulation and heart must be adjusted to a steady rhythm of work in order to regenerate.

Nightly rest must be respected above all: It must be abundant. More sleep before midnight is necessary. Breaking this rule for several nights frequently causes relapses. Rising early and going for a walk in the early morning serves to stimulate respiration and circulation.

Midday rest: After lunch, disrobe and go to bed for a whole hour.

Two small walks per day, e.g., early morning and afternoon, or in the evening before going to sleep should become a habit. Weekend hikes with gradually increased activity, but without strenous performance, are recommended.

Respiration: Respiration enables one to consciously affect the regulation. Steady, deep breathing can achieve a considerable lowering of blood pressure when weakened pressure regulation is involved. Practice several times per day, especially morning and evening; while maintaining a natural posture, breathe out with a completely relaxed, comfortable and prolonged expiration to the point where inspiration again occurs spontaneously.

Relaxation: Concentrating on one's entire weight, one tries to feel it and fully rest it on the bed or couch, until a healthy warmth spreads into the limbs as a sign of relaxation. Practice this repeatedly until it begins to occur easily.

Skin care: In the morning brush with a dry brush and wash with cool water.

Simple hydrotherapy: A cold abdominal compress at night is a simple and effective aid in the cure of a full and heavy abdomen. The compress causes blood pressure to fall markedly during the night, and healthful relaxation occurs. Arm baths of increasing temperatures simply and effectively relieve blood pressure and heart: The arms are immersed in 96°F water to the middle of the upper arm, and the temperature is raised slowly to 113°F—over at least 10 minutes—by adding hot water until mild sweating occurs. After 10 minutes more, rest lightly covered. Do same for the feet, immersed up to mid-calf, or with arms and feet together.

Sun: Sun baths are very valuable, when started with a 5-minute session, slowly increasing to 15 minutes for each side of the body. The head should be kept in the shade. Afterwards, light clothing and rest.

Psychic conditions: As far as possible try to avoid discussions and situations which lead to irritation and tension. Urgently avoid late-night parties and try to find one hour a day in which to be alone to organize thoughts and feelings, giving conscious attention to constructive and happy thoughts.

Medicines: Blood pressure effective rutin-preparations, mistletoe extracts and ergot preparations, as well as lemon balm, valerian, and hop extracts against nervous tension will be prescribed by the physician when necessary.

II. Recipes

MUESLI

The original recipe for muesli, as it was first worked out by Dr. Bircher-Benner, should be considered a prescription rather than a recipe. If closely followed it will not only provide the best balance of essential nutrients, but experience has also shown that people will not become tired of it, if regularly taken once or twice per day—something which may easily happen if richer and more elaborate versions are offered.

Any apple which is juicy, tart and white-fleshed is recommended. A combination of eating and cooking apples often yields the best results. For example, any of the following, alone or in combination: Cortland, McIntoch, Rhode Island Greening, Northern Spy, Winesap, Jonathan, Gravenstein.

Later on in the season, when home-grown apples tend to become dry and tasteless, their flavor can be improved by the addition, just before serving, of some freshly grated orange or lemon peel, orange juice or rose hip purée.

The orange and lemon peel must come from fruits that have not been sprayed with DDT or Diphenyl.

1. Apple Muesli

1 tbsp. rolled oats
3 tbsp. water, cold
1 tbsp. lemon juice

1 tbsp. sweetened condensed milk or unsweetened
1 large apple (or 2-3 small ones)
1 tbsp. grater filberts or almonds (hazelnuts)

The oats must be soaked beforehand for 12 hrs. (It is not necessary to soak the quick-cooking varieties. The amount of water used remains the same.)

Mix lemon juice and condensed milk to a smooth cream. Wash apples, wipe with cloth and remove tops, cores and any blemishes. Using a two-way or Bircher grater, grate apple into mixture, stirring frequently to prevent discoloring. (Grating should be done immediately before serving.) Sprinkle nuts over the finished dish and serve immediately.

Instead of 1 tbsp. rolled oats, the following can be used: 1 tsp. rolled oats, previously soaked, and 1 tsp. cereal grains. These should be soaked in water 24 hrs., then, rinsed through a sieve and in cold water, and used either whole, coarsely ground, crushed or prepared in electric blender. Alternatively, cereal flakes such as wheat, rice, barley, rye, millet, buckwheat or soya or dried wheat flakes (possibly mixed with yeast flakes for vitamin B) may be used. Most of these are obtainable at health food stores or leading grocers.

2. Apple Muesli with Almond Puree

(Muesli without animal protein; for vegetarians and in cases of allergy.)

1 tbsp. rolled oats soaked for 12 hrs. in 3 tbsp. water
1 tbsp. almond purée diluted in 3 tbsp. water
1 tbsp. lemon juice
1 tbsp. honey
1 large apple
2 tbsp. grated filberts or almonds

Stir constantly until the mixture becomes emulsified. Prepare and add the apple as in Basic Recipe, no. 1. Sprinkle grated nuts over the prepared dish.

3. Apple Muesli with Yogurt

(Diet when milk is not tolerated, promotes digestion; tart, not filling.)

>   1 tbsp. rolled oats
>   3 tbsp. water
>   3 tbsp. yogurt
>   1 tbsp. honey or 1-1/2 tbsp. raw sugar
>   1 tbsp. lemon juice
>   7 oz apple
>   1 tbsp. grated hazelnuts or almonds

Soak the oats for 12 hrs. Mix the yogurt, lemon juice, and honey into a smooth sauce. Prepare the apple as in the Basic Recipe, no. 1. Sprinkle chopped nuts over the prepared dish.

4. Muesli with Berries or Stone Fruit

(Especially rich in vitamin C.)

>   1/2 lb. strawberries, raspberries, or blueberries, red
>   currants, blackberries, or
>   1/2 lb. peaches, apricots or plums

For berries: Select, wash and hull berries. Crush with fork or wooden spoon.

For stone fruit: Select, wash and stone. Chop up or reduce to pulp in electric blender. Prepare sauce as in Basic Recipe, no. 1.

5. Muesli with Mixed Fruits

>   Strawberries and raspberries
>   Strawberries and apple
>   Blackberries and apple

Apple with finely cut oranges or tangerine slices
Apple and banana
Plums, peaches or apricots, etc.*

For preparation of the sauce refer to Basic Recipe, no. 1.

6. Muesli with Dried Fruits

If situations arise when muesli must be prepared with dried fruits (apples, apricots, prunes), 4 oz. dried fruits can be washed per portion, soaked in cold water for 12 hrs. and put through a mincer. Add this purée to the mixture in Basic Recipe, no. 1.

Care must be taken that the dried fruit is of good quality, without preservatives or bleaching agents, otherwise troublesome gastric and intestinal disturbances may result. Although this dried-fruit muesli is also of dietetic value, it, of course, lacks the therapeutic potency of fresh-fruit muesli and thus, is not a permanent replacement for the latter.

RAW VEGETABLES

The following four principles must be observed in the preparation of raw vegetables:

1. Freshness

The ideal vegetables are sun-ripened, organically grown, compost fertilized, from one's own garden.

Raw vegetables should, if possible, be prepared just before they are intended to be eaten, so that no wilting and loss of juice takes place. After they have been chopped, grated or shredded they should not be exposed to the air for too long but should be mixed immediately with the dressing to prevent oxidizing.

---

* Apricots and prunes should be avoided by those suffering from stomach or intestinal ailments.

2. Quality

Leaf and roof vegetables should be young, tender and of good color. They should have been grown, whenever possible, on soil fertilized with compost and be free of plant diseases. This is specially important in the case of invalid diet.

3. Thorough Cleaning

The instructions given below on the cleaning of vegetables must be followed exactly, to get rid of any worms and to avoid infection with colibacilli.

Compost-grown vegetables, and those grown without chemical or animal manure, do not contain any worm eggs.

4. Well-Balanced Mixtures

Whenever possible, every raw vegetable dish should combine roots-fruit-leaves. Invalid diet, in particular, should always include green leaves. The dressing used for the same raw vegetable salad should also be varied as much as possible.

Bright and harmonious colors make the salad dishes more attractive and increase the pleasure of eating.

Herbs, radishes and young carrots, etc., are effective as decorations when, for special occasions, a more festive air is wanted. Not more than three raw vegetables, however, should be served for any single daily salad, more attention being paid to variety during the course of the day. Too much variety can have a bad effect on the digestion.

Cleaning Leafy Vegetables: Boston lettuce, Romaine lettuce, endive, kale, white cabbage, red cabbage, etc., separate the leaves, remove brown and imperfect parts and leave to soak for 1 hr. in slightly salted water (1 handful to about 6 qts. water). Rinse several times, if possible washing each leaf separately under the tap. Drain well in wire basket or clean cloth.

Special care must be taken with the preparation and

washing of corn salad or lamb's lettuce, spinach, dandelion, lettuce, cress, Brussels sprouts, and similar small leafy salads. Remove any little roots and tough parts and rinse thoroughly.

Halve chicory, remove outer leaves and wash well.

Cleaning Root Vegetables: Carrots, beetroots, turnips, radishes, kohlrabi, celeriac and salsify. Scrub roots with a brush under running water. Peel and put immediately into cold water to which salt and lemon juice have been added (half a lemon or squeezed out peel to about 6 qts. water), so that vegetables do not lose their fresh color.

Cleaning of Vegetable Fruits: Tomatoes, cucumbers, zucchini, green and red peppers. Wash and if necessary, peel and cut up into small pieces.

Peel cucumbers starting from the center, working towards the ends. Cut off bitter ends. Tender cucumbers need not be peeled.

Use only very young, tender zucchini for salad; do not peel. Green peppers are less sharp than the red variety. Cut peppers in half and remove the seeds, score thick parts and soak in water if too sharp.

Cut cauliflower into quarters, remove imperfect parts, scrape stalk lightly and put into salt water. Scrape celery and cut away tough part. Halve leeks, remove bad parts and rinse thoroughly. Halve fennel and wash.

Special Methods of Cleaning: If there is any doubt as to the growing and hygienic handling of any fruit or vegetables, or their freedom from bacteria, the following methods of cleaning must be observed:

1. In order to destroy any worm eggs and insects, put vegetables into a diluted salt solution (1 handful cooking salt to about 6 qts. water). The salt solution dissolves the protein layer by which the worm eggs are attached and subsequent rinsing of the vegetables removes them.

2. Bacteria, colibacilli and fungi, which are not harmful to healthy people, particularly in northern countries, can be removed with citric acid or vinegar. The vegetables, particularly leafy ones, should be left in a

solution of 2 oz. citric acid to about 2 pts. water for
15 min. Rinse well afterwards under running water.
If the citric acid solution is strained and set aside, it
can be used three of four times.
3. Put root vegetables and vegetable fruits in a colander
or sieve and dip into boiling water for ten seconds.
The outer layer is thus freed of any bacteria while the
vegetables remain raw inside.
4. Vegetable and fruit juices can be practically freed of
bacteria if lemon juice is added (one-fifth of the total
quantity of juice).
5. To prevent any danger of amoebic infection in the
tropics, dip the prepared vegetables into a chloride of
lime solution (1/6 oz. to 2 pts. water), then wash
well in boiled water, to remove all traces of it.

Various Methods of Cutting up Vegetables

Boston lettuce, Redleaf lettuce, lamb's lettuce,
  dandelion, cress—leave whole or halve largest leaves
Romaine lettuce, endive, chicory—cut into 1/4 in.
  strips
Spinach, leeks, peppers, celery, fennel—shred
Kale, white and red cabbage—shred finely
Carrots, beetroots, celeriac, white radishes, salsify,
  kohlrabi—grate with Bircher grater or a coarse
  grater
Cucumbers, red radishes, cauliflower, zucchini—
  slice very finely or grate with Bircher grater

SALAD DRESSINGS

7. French Dressing

1 tbsp. oil
Some onion or garlic
1 tsp. fresh or a pinch of dried herbs
1 tsp. lemon juice

Mix all ingredients together thoroughly.

8. Mayonnaise Dressing with Soy Flour Instead of Egg

2 level tbsp. soy flour
6 tbsp. water
7 oz. oil
3 tbsp. lemon juice
Some onion
1 tsp. fresh or a pinch dried herbs

Mix the soy flour and water to a smooth paste. Add oil and lemon juice alternately, very slowly, then whisk well. Mix in onion and herbs.

9. Yogurt Dressing

2-3 tbsp. yogurt
Few drops lemon juice
1 tsp. fresh or 1/4 tsp. dried herbs
Some onion, garlic (opt.)

Whisk all ingredients thoroughly together.

10. Almond Purée or Sauce

1 tbsp. almond purée
3 tbsp. water
1 tsp. lemon juice
Some onions, garlic (opt.)
1 tsp. fresh or 1/4 tsp. dried herbs

Add water and mix all ingredients together slowly and thoroughly.

The Following Raw Vegetables†

11. Boston Lettuce	Use whole leaves
12. Redleaf Lettuce	Use whole leaves
13. Endive	Cut in 1/2-in. strips
14. Romaine Lettuce	Cut in 1/2-in. strips
15. Lamb's Lettuce	Use whole leaves
16. Cresses	Use whole leaves
17. Spinach	Cut in 1/4-in. strips
18. Cabbage: white cabbage, sauerkraut, savoy, Brussels sprouts, Chinese cabbage	Shred finely
19. Tomatoes	Slice or dice
20. Cucumbers	Slice finely
21. Fennel	Slice finely and chop
22. Peppers	Shred finely
23. White Radishes	Slice or grate
24. Red Radishes	Slice
25. Celery	Shred finely
26. Squash or Zucchini	Slice finely or grate roughly
27. Carrots	Grate finely
28. Celeriac	Grate finely
29. Beetroots	Grate finely or roughly
30. Cauliflower	Separate florets, grate stalks
31. Chicory and Belgian Endives	Cut in 1/2-in. strips
32. Jerusalem Artichokes	Grate
33. Kohlrabi	Grate and chop finely
34. Red cabbage	Shred or grate finely

Note: For cleaning and cutting of vegetables, see Raw Vegetables, p. 34.

† A moderate quantity of chives, parsley and onion may be added to every dish of raw vegetables.

French dressing		Chives, onion
French dressing		Chives, onion
French dressing		Chives, onion, parsley
French dressing		Sweet basil, marjoram
French dressing		Onion
French dressing		Onion
French dressing	or almond purée sauce	Peppermint
French dressing	or almond purée sauce	Lovage, savory, thyme, dill
French dressing		Basil, thyme, dill
French dressing		Dill
French dressing	or soya mayonnaise	Onion, chives
French dressing	or almond purée sauce	Chives
French dressing		Chives
French dressing		Chives
French dressing		Onion, chives
French dressing	or almond purée sauce	Dill, basil, borage
French dressing		Marjoram, lovage
French dressing		Basil, thyme
French dressing		Lovage, thyme, caraway seeds
Almond purée sauce	or soya mayonnaise	Basil, marjoram, walnuts
French dressing		Tarragon, marjoram
Almond purée sauce		Thyme, lemon balm
French dressing	or almond purée sauce	Thyme, lovage
Almond purée sauce		Some grated apple, caraway seeds, lovage

35. Mixed Raw Vegetables

Chicory with diced tomato (French dressing)
Peppers and fennel (French dressing)
Fennel, chicory and diced tomato (Soya mayonnaise)
Fennel and carrots (French dressing)
Cauliflower and carrots (Almond purée sauce)
Tomato and peppers (French dressing)

36. Stuffed Raw Tomatoes

With cucumber and French dressing
With celeriac and French dressing or almond purée
    sauce
With cauliflower and almond purée sauce
With white cabbage and French dressing

37. Sprouted Cereal Grains

(Especially high in vitamins E and B. Good for all-around fitness.)
Wheat, rye, oats, barley (whole grains).

1st day
evening: Wash grains in sieve under running water and put in a bowl. Cover with water. Keep at room temperature near stove or radiator.

2nd day
morning: Rinse and spread out to dry on a flat plate. Keep at room temperature near stove or radiator.

3rd day
morning: Rinse and spread out to dry on a plate.
evening: Place in a bowl and cover with water. Keep at room temperature near stove or radiator.

The grains should have 1/2-3/4 in. long sprouts.

38. Special Child's Cereal

Cracked cereal grains, soaked and mixed in blender with bananas, honey and water

Sauerkraut

Sauerkraut is a very valuable raw vegetable, particularly in winter, as it is rich in vitamin C. It is easier to digest when raw than when cooked. If sauerkraut is cooked occasionally, its flavor and digestibility can be improved by adding finely cut fresh sauerkraut.

Sauerkraut Salad

Loosen sauerkraut and cut up, mix with some caraway seeds (or ground caraway), 3-4 crushed juniper berries, finely sliced onion and shredded apple. Mix thoroughly with the juice of 1 lemon and 2 tbsp. olive oil. Serve with corn salad (or watercress) and with any variety of uncooked root salads.

JUICES

Juices are uncooked food in a form which is liquidized by some mechanical means. They are meant to be special enrichment to the diet and are of considerable value in cases where roughage (cellulose) must be avoided, or in the case of gastrointestinal conditions.

It should, however, be realized that the whole fruit is, always of greater value, and, in the long run, cannot be replaced by juices. As soon as permissible, a return should therefore be made to whole fruit and raw vegetables.

For cleaning, refer to introductory section on Raw Vege-

Note: For salt-free diets, take care to buy unsalted sauerkraut.

tables. Juice extractors are obtainable for squeezing out
the fruit and vegetable juices. These include the small hand
press, the juice-extracting attachment of an electric food
mixer, or electric blender. If the hand press is used, the
fruit or vegetables must be first cut up.

39. Fruit Juices

Serve immediately after extracting. Delay of any kind
causes loss in value.

39a. Unmixed Fruit Juices (without any addition):

Oranges, tangerines, grapefruit, apples, pears, grapes,
strawberries, raspberries, red currants, blueberries,
peaches, apricots, plums

39b. Mixed Fruit Juices:

Orange, tangerine, grapefruit, or berry juice with apple
juice
Berry juice with peach, apricot or plum juice
Bananas, mashed and whisked, with orange, peach or
apricot juice

Additional ingredients as required or prescribed:
Lemon juice, raw sugar, honey, pure fruit concentrates,
yogurt, almond purée, cream of linseed, rice, or barley (for
gastrointestinal conditions).

40. Vegetable Juices

Served fresh, they have a high vitamin and mineral content. Each juice has its own special value (see chapter on
mineral substances and vitamins in the Bircher-Benner
cookbook, *Eating Your Way to Health,* Penguin).

40a. Unmixed Vegetable Juices:

Tomatoes, carrots, beetroot, white radishes, cabbage, celeriac, potatoes, all leaf, root and tuberous vegetables

40b. Mixed Vegetable Juices:

In our experience, the best mixtures are:
Carrots, tomatoes, spinach (in equal proportions)
Tomatoes and carrots
Tomatoes and spinach

Other mixtures (and vegetable cocktails) can be combined according to individual taste.

For a change, add to the mixture before extracting, some sorrel, tender nettles, chives, parsley, tender young celery or celeriac leaves or root. Other leaf vegetables which may be added include: white or green cabbage, Boston lettuce, endive, lamb's lettuce, dandelion. In spring, dandelion, sorrel and nettle juice are suggested to cleanse the blood.

Additional supplementary ingredients
Per glass (about 5-7 oz.):
1 tbsp. yogurt, some lemon juice, fruit concentrate; or cream of linseed, rice or barley.

40c. Potato Juice:

Use well-cleaned, if necessary peeled, potatoes, use no unripe, greenish or sprouting ones
Prepare like carrot juice. Does not taste very pleasant, but may be suggested by a doctor.

41. Cereal Cream as Supplement to Juices

One-third of cereal cream can be added to raw juices. It neutralizes tart fruit flavors.

Note: If there is no opportunity to prepare juices at home, high-value bottled grape-, fruit- and vegetable juices can be obtained at health food stores.

41a. Cream of rice or barley:

> 1 heaping tsp. rice or barley flour
> 7 oz. water

Mix flour with some cold water. Bring to a boil. Cook for 5 min., stirring constantly. Allow to cool.

41b. Cream of linseed:

> 1 tbsp. linseed
> 7 oz. water

Wash linsed in a sieve under running water. Boil in the water for 10 minutes. Strain and allow to cool.

The daily quantity of cereal cream for gastrointestinal patients can be prepared at one time, then put into a thermos flask and added to each freshly prepared raw juice as required.

VARIETIES OF MILK

42. Almond Milk

(A vegetable protein-fat-food; mucilaginous; soothing.)

> 1 tbsp. almond purée
> 1 tsp. honey
> 3/4 cup water (or 3/4 cup water and 1/4 cup fruit
>   juice to produce slight thickening)

Mix almond purée and honey together with whisk. Add water drop by drop continually whisking or stirring well.

43. Almond Milk from Fresh Almonds

(Especially easy to digest.)

  1-1/2 tbsp. peeled almonds (do not use bitter
     almonds)
  1 tsp. honey
  3/4 cup water

Mix in electric blender or mixer. Strain if necessary.

44. Pine Kernel Milk

(Extremely rich in easily digestible fat and vegetable protein.)

  1-1/2 tbsp. washed pine kernels
  1 tsp. honey
  3/4 cup water

Prepare like Almond Milk.

45. Sesame Milk

  1 cup water (hot or cold, according to taste)
  1 level tbsp. sesame purée
  1 tsp. honey
  1 tsp. lemon juice

Mix the purée, honey and lemon juice with a wire whisk while adding water drop by drop until the consistency of milk.

46. Sesame Cream

Prepare like Sesame Milk, adding less water; use with fruit desserts and as a substitute for cream.

47. Sesame Frappé

Prepare like Sesame Milk or Sesame Cream, adding fruit juice, fruit concentrates, etc.

48. Soy Milk

1 cup grated soy beans
7 cups water
water to mix
1 tbsp. sugar

Wash and dry soy beans, grate in a nutmill or an electric blender. Soak soy beans for 2 hrs. Boil for 20 min. in soaking water, stirring constantly. Rub through a sieve. Add water until purée has the consistency of cow's milk. Add sugar and allow to cool.

49. Yogurt I

Yogurt is the purest, most efficacious and easily digestible food for supplying milk protein. It stimulates the digestion.
The simplest way to make yogurt at home is with an electric yogurt maker. Manufacturer's directions must be followed closely.

50. Yogurt II

4 cups milk
3 oz. yogurt

Bring milk to a boil. Cool to 100°F. Whisk yogurt together with milk. Pour into a glass receptacle. Cover with cheesecloth and a lid. Cover with blanket or pillows or put in very low oven. Leave warm for 24 hrs. Store in refrigerator until use.

Commercial yogurt can be used if a good quality can be obtained from a dairy or a health food store.

51. Butter, Vegetable Fats, Oils

Fresh butter (unsalted): (Only when allowed) to enrich dishes, and in most diet recipes

Health food store vegetable margarine: Vegetable fat emulsion from natural solid fats like coconut oil or palm seed oil combined with the largest possible amount of liquid oils and seed oils—especially sunflower oil. Fine, nut-like flavor, very useful for cooking and serving

Nut and Almond Purée: Prepared from pure hazelnuts and almonds as a spread and used like fresh butter on vegetables, potatoes, rice and pasta

Sunflower oil, linseed oil, cornseed oil, olive oil: Carefully processed, very valuable because of their purity as fats and more easily digestible for most people than heated butter.

Note: Other cold-pressed vegetable fats and oils, available in health food stores, are also recommended for health-food cuisine.

SOUPS

In our soup and vegetable recipes we use large amounts of vegetable stock. In a small household where fresh vegetable stock cannot be prepared daily, water can be used with liquid yeast extract or salt-free vegetable bouillon cubes. Add margarine, or milk, if allowed, to improve flavor.

Health food store yeast extracts are very rich in vitamin B (rich in glutathione and lecithin).

Note: *Add 1 pinch salt to all cooked recipes (except sweet dishes).*

52. Vegetable Broth

This recipe is for 4 servings. All others are for 1 serving.

Choose vegetables in season, for instance, celery, carrots, some cabbage or kohlrabi, leeks, tomatoes, celeriac and onions. The tougher but still sound parts may also be used, as well as potato peel.

    1 tbsp. vegetable margarine
    1 onion
    2 carrots
    1 cup diced celeriac
    Cabbage leaves, spinach or beet leaves
    3-4 qts. cold water
    Lovage, basil or other fresh or dried herbs
    1/2 bay leaf
    Salt

Melt fat. Halve onion, with skin, and brown cut surface in fat. Cut vegetables in small pieces. Add to the onion and steam gently for at least 1/4 hr., covered with a lid. Add cold water, simmer for 2 hrs. Strain. Season according to taste.

53. Vegetable Bouillon

    1-1/2 cups vegetable stock
    Salt-free yeast extract to taste
    1/2 oz. vegetable cooking fat

Season with parsley or chives, and freshly chopped herbs. Pour hot vegetable stock over the fat and seasonings.

Additions to Soup

54. Butter Dumplings

1/2 tbsp. butter,
1 tbsp. flour
2 tbsp. milk, hot
1/2 egg (beaten)

Melt butter and sauté flour in it. Add milk and beat until mixture leaves sides of the pan. Mix beaten egg with hot paste. Scoop out small dumplings with teaspoon, add to boiling stock and simmer for 5 min. Season with lovage, basil, parsley, chives, marjoram or possibly nutmeg.

55. Farina Dumplings

(When egg is permitted.)

1/2 oz. vegetable margarine or butter
1-1/2 tbsp. fine farina
1/2-1 egg

Blend fat. Mix in other ingredients and let stand for 1/2 hr. Scoop out dumplings with the tip of a teaspoon, drop into boiling vegetable stock and simmer for 15 to 20 min. Season with nutmeg and marjoram.

56. Tapioca Soup with Vegetables

1/2 oz. tapioca
2 cups vegetable stock
1/2 tbsp. vegetable margarine
1 small carrot
1 small stick of celery root
1 small leek

Add tapioca to simmering broth. Cut vegetables into small cubes or strips. Sauté the vegetables in the fat, add to stock and cook for 1/2 hr. Season with salt-free yeast extract, parsley, chives.

57. Clear Rice Soup

1/2 tbsp. vegetable margarine
Some chopped onion
Small carrot, thinly sliced
Some celery root, thinly sliced
Leek, thinly sliced
2 cups vegetable stock
1 tbsp. rice

Melt fat, sauté the vegetables. Add rice and stock. Simmer for 1/2 hr.

58. Thick Rice Soup

1/2 tbsp. vegetable margarine
Celery root, thinly sliced
Small carrot, thinly sliced
Leek, thinly sliced
1 tbsp. rice
1/2 tbsp. flour
2-1/2 cups vegetable stock or water
Chives

Melt fat. Sauté vegetables. Add rice and sauté together. Sprinkle flour over all. Add stock and seasoning, cook for 30 min. Add chives to finished soup.

Season with salt-free yeast extract, lovage, parsley, basil, marjoram.

59. Creamed Rice Soup

1 tbsp. rice flour
1/4 tbsp. wheat flour
4 tbsp. milk
2-1/2 cups vegetable stock
1/2 tbsp. vegetable margarine
1 tbsp. milk

Bring stock to boil. Blend rice, milk and flour. Cook for 1/2 hr. in the broth. Add fat and milk to the finished soup. Season with chives, marjoram, perhaps nutmeg or caraway.

60. Herb Soup

1 tbsp. whole-wheat flour
1/2 cup milk
2 cups vegetable stock
1/4 oz. butter (opt.)

Mix flour with some milk and stir into simmering vegetable stock. Cook for 1/4 hr. Place butter into the soup tureen and stir in the cooked soup. Season with lovage, marjoram, chives, basil, tarragon, possibly nutmeg or caraway.

61. Soy Soup

1/2 tbsp. vegetable margarine
Some onion
1 tbsp. whole-wheat flour
1/2 tbsp. soy flour
1/2 tomato, peeled and diced
2 cups vegetable stock

Melt fat and sauté onion, adding wheat and soy flour. Add tomato and stock. Cook for 1/4 hr. Season with basil, marjoram, possibly rosemary, chives, parsley.

62. Cream of Oat Soup

1/2 tbsp. flour
2 tbsp. rolled oats
2-1/2 cups vegetable stock
Some celery root*
1/2 tbsp. vegetable fat
2 tbsp. milk

Melt fat, brown flour and oats lightly. Add vegetable stock and celery root. Cook for 1 hr. Strain. Add milk to the tureen. Season with yeast extract, chives, possibly nutmeg, caraway, or chopped dried mushrooms.

63. Oat Groats Soup

1/2 tbsp. vegetable margarine
2 tbsp. oat groats
Some chopped onion
3 cups water or vegetable stock
1/2 cup milk
Some celery root*
Yeast extract

Lightly brown the oats and onions in fat. Add stock, milk, and celery root. Cook for 1 hr. Add yeast extract to the tureen. Season with chives, parsley, marjoram or borage.

---

* Omit, when on a strict salt-free diet.

64. Green Spelt Soup

1/2 tbsp. vegetable margarine
Some onion chopped
1 tbsp. leek, cut fine
Celery root, diced small
1-2 tbsp. green spelt (whole or cracked) soaked for
    12 hrs. in 1/2 cup water
2 cups vegetable stock

Melt fat and sauté onion. Add leek and celery root and sauté together. Add to the green spelt. Add the stock and cook for 1 to 1-1/2 hrs. Season with chopped lovage (or perhaps celery herbs). Strain the soup or run through blender, if necessary.

65. Vaudois Farina Soup

1/2 tbsp. vegetable margarine
1 tbsp. farina
1/2 tbsp. whole-wheat flour
2 tbsp. cabbage, finely shredded
2-1/2 cups vegetable stock
1/4 oz. fresh butter

Melt margarine. Sauté farina and flour in it. Add cabbage and saute until cabbage loses its crispness. Pour in the stock and cook altogether for 1/2 hr. Put butter into tureen and pour soup over it. Season with salt-free yeast extract, finely chopped caraway, or nutmeg, 1 clove, lovage, basil, marjoram, parsley, chives.

66. Browned Whole-wheat Soup

1 tbsp. whole-wheat flour
1 tbsp. flour
2-1/2 cups vegetable stock, cold
1/4 onion
Some caraway seeds
1/2 oz. butter
1 tbsp. grated cheese (opt.)

Roast flour until hazelnut brown, then cool. Slowly add the cold vegetable stock, stirring the flour until smooth. Add onion, caraway seeds and cook for 1/2 hr. Put butter and cheese into the tureen and pour soup over it. Season with bay leaf, or nutmeg, clove, marjoram, yeast extract.

67. Tomato Soup I

1/2 tbsp. vegetable margarine
Some onion
2 tbsp. small carrots
Celery root*
Leek
Clove of garlic
Some rosemary
1 tomato
1 tbsp. flour
2-1/2 cups vegetable stock
1/4 oz. butter
Tomato purée (opt.)

Cut onion, carrots, leek and garlic finely and sauté. Add tomato. Sprinkle with flour. Add stock, cook for 1/2 hr. and strain. Season with a clove, chives, laurel; add butter before serving.

Note: A tbsp, of rice or tapioca may be added, or croutons.

---

* Omit, when on a strict salt-free diet.

68. Tomato Soup II

4 ripe summer tomatoes
1 tsp. of lemon juice or sugar (opt.)
2 tbsp. yogurt

Slice the tomatoes, cook quickly and strain. Add lemon juice and yogurt; serve soup hot or cold.

69. Carrot Soup

1/2 tbsp. vegetable margarine
Some onion
1 sliced carrot
1-1/2 tbsp. flour
2 cups vegetable stock
1/2 cup milk
1 tsp. caraway
Celery or lovage

Melt fat, sauté onions and carrots. Sprinkle flour over mixture and sauté lightly. Add stock and milk. Cook for 1/2 hr. Strain. Season with sugar browned in butter, rosemary or marjoram.

70. Spinach Soup*

1/2 tbsp. vegetable margarine
Some onion
1/2 clove of garlic
1-1/2 tbsp. flour
2 cups vegetable stock
1/2 cup milk
1 small cup spinach
Some peppermint leaves
Nutmeg

* Omit, when on a strict salt-free diet.

Melt fat and sauté onion, garlic and flour in it. Add stock and cook for 20 min. Add raw, finely chopped spinach and peppermint leaves to the finished soup and do not allow to boil again. Put nutmeg into tureen and pour soup over it. Season with parsley, chives, salt-free yeast extract, or sage leaves.

71. Cauliflower Soup

1/2 tbsp. vegetable margarine
1-1/2 tbsp. flour
Some cauliflower florets
2 cups vegetable stock
1/4 bay leaf
Basil (very little)
2 tbsp. milk (opt.)

Cook cauliflower florets separately. Cut uncooked stalks into small pieces. Melt fat and sauté flour in it. Add cut-up stalks and sauté together. Add stock, salt, bay leaf and basil and cook for 3/4 hr. Strain. Put cooked florets and milk into soup shortly before serving. Season with yeast extract, parsley, chives, tarragon or nutmeg.

72. Chervil Soup

1/2 tbsp. vegetable margarine
Some onion
1 medium potato, diced
1/2 tbsp. flour
2 cups vegetable stock
1 tbsp. chervil, chopped
2 tbsp. milk (opt.)

Melt fat. Sauté onion. Add diced potatoes and sauté, sprinkling flour over the mixture. Add stock and cook for

1/2 hr. Strain. Place chervil and milk into tureen and pour soup over.

73. Spring Soup

1/2 tbsp. vegetable margarine
1 tbsp. flour
2 cups water or vegetable stock
Some onion
1 tbsp. young carrot, some spinach leaves*
1/2 cup milk

Melt fat, brown flour lightly, add water and cook for 1/2 hr. Chop onion, herbs and vegetables. Add to soup and simmer for a few minutes. Add milk and serve. Season with lovage, sorrel, wood nettle or dandelion leaves.

74. Cream of Leek Soup

1/2 tbsp. vegetable margarine
1/4 leek, cut-up coarsely
1-1/2 tbsp. flour
2-1/2 cups vegetable stock
2 tbsp. milk

Melt fat and sauté leek in it till tender. Sprinkle flour over it. Add stock and cook 1/2-3/4 hrs. Strain. Put milk into tureen and add soup. Season with salt-free yeast extract, nutmeg.

---

* Omit spinach, when on a strict salt-free diet.

75. Onion Soup

1/2 tbsp. vegetable margarine
1 onion, cut in strips
1 tbsp. flour
2 cups water or vegetable stock
2 tbsp. milk (opt.)

Melt fat and sauté onion in it till tender. Sprinkle flour over it and sauté some more. Add and cook 1/2 hr. (Strain if preferred.) Put milk into tureen and add soup. Season with yeast extract, basil, nutmeg.

76. Potato Soup with Leek

1/2 tbsp. vegetable margarine
1/2 leek, cut in strips
1/2 tbsp. flour
2 cups vegetable stock
1 medium potato, cut into small pieces
2 tbsp. milk (opt.)

Sauté leek well in fat. Sprinkle flour over it. Add stock and potato. Simmer for a few minutes. Milk may be added to the tureen before serving. Season with yeast extract, marjoram, basil, dried mushrooms.

77. Brown Potato Soup

1 tbsp. flour
2 cups water
1 medium potato, sliced
1/2 tbsp. grated cheese
Some fresh butter

Roast flour to a chestnut brown. Slowly add cold water and mix well. Add potato, and cook until soft. Put cheese into tureen and pour soup over it. Season with caraway, or marjoram.

78. Cabbage and Potato Soup

1/2 tbsp. vegetable margarine
Some onion
1 small cabbage, finely shredded
1/2 tbsp. flour
1 potato, sliced
2 cups water
2 tbsp. milk

Melt fat and sauté onion. Add cabbage and sauté gently until soft. Sprinkle flour over the mixture and sauté together for a short time. Add potatoes, water and cook for 1/2 hr. Put milk into tureen or soup bowls and pour soup over it.

79. Green Bean Soup

1/2 tbsp. vegetable margarine
1/2 clove of garlic
2 oz. beans, sliced diagonally

Melt fat. Sauté chopped garlic in it. Add sliced beans and sauté. Add water and cook until soft. Add to Cream Soup, Recipe no. 59. Season with marjoram, thyme, savory.

80. Yellow Pea Soup

2 oz. yellow peas
1-1/4 cups water
1 small potato
1-1/4 cups vegetable stock
1/2 tbsp. vegetable margarine
Some onion, chopped
2 tbsp. leek
1 small carrot
1 piece of celeriac (Leave out in strict
    sodium-free diets)
1/2 tbsp. flour (opt.)
2 tbsp. milk (opt.)
1 tbsp. sautéed bread cubes

Soak peas in the water for 12 hours. Cook peas and potato in soaking water for 1 to 1-1/2 hrs. Strain and add stock. Melt fat and sauté the onion and finely shredded vegetables. Sprinkle flour over the mixture and sauté. Stir in strained soup, gradually. Cook gently for 20 min. Put milk into tureen or soup bowls and pour soup over it. Serve with sautéed bread cubes. Season with parsley, chives.

81. Minestrone Soup

(Not for strict sodium-free diets.)

1/2 tbsp. vegetable margarine
Some onion
2 tbsp. leek
A few celery root leaves
1/2 plateful spinach or beet leaves
3 cups water or vegetable stock
1 tbsp. lovage or thyme
1/2 clove of garlic
1/2 oz. whole-wheat pasta, or rice
1/4 oz. butter

Sauté finely sliced onion and leek. Add chopped greens and braise. Add stock and cook for 1/2 hr. Add butter to enrich flavor. Season with parsley, basil, chives.

COOKED VEGETABLES

82. Chopped Spinach

Select spinach carefully, throw away the thickest stalks. Wash thoroughly.

1 cup vegetable stock
7 oz. spinach
1/2 tbsp. vegetable margarine
A little chopped onion
Some fresh garlic
1 tbsp. flour
1 cup raw spinach

Place chopped spinach without water in saucepan, cover tightly, cook very briefly over low heat. Melt fat, sauté onion and garlic while adding flour. Add stock and cook to thicken. Add spinach with the cooking juice. Finely mince raw spinach and add before serving. Season with peppermint leaves, sage, fresh butter.

83. Spinach, Whole Leaves

1/2 tbsp. vegetable margarine or oil
Some onion, chopped
10 oz. spinach
1 tbsp. pine kernels
1 tbsp. raisins
Some vegetable stock (opt.)

Pick over spinach, remove thickest stalks, wash thoroughly. Melt fat and sauté onion until golden. Add spinach, pine kernels, raisins and stock and cook over low flame until tender, uncovered. Season with peppermint leaves, sage, parsley, or cover with hot butter. (Winter spinach should be blanched for a short time before use.)

84. Baked Romaine Lettuce

1 Romaine lettuce
4 cups water
1/2 tbsp. vegetable margarine
1/2 cup vegetable stock
2 tbsp. milk (opt.)

Halve and wash the lettuce. Cook gently in salted water. When partly cooked but still firm put into a colander to drain. Place in a baking dish. Melt fat, sauté onion in it until golden and pour over lettuce. Add stock and bake in medium oven 30-40 minutes. Add milk 5 min. before serving.

85. Baked Endive

1 large head endive

Prepare as for Romaine lettuce, Recipe no. 84.

86. Chicory or Belgian Endive

1 head chicory, prepared or 2 Belgian endives
1/2 tbsp. vegetable margarine
2 tbsp. milk
1 tbsp. vegetable stock
Some butter

Make crosswise incision in chicory or endive stalks. Heat cooking fat in a heavy saucepan and put in vegetable in layers. Add milk and stock, cover and cook gently for 1/2 hr. Add butter to the cooled dish. Season with marjoram, onion, thyme, apple.

87. Stalks of Spinach Beet

3 stalks spinach beet, prepared
1/2 tbsp. vegetable margarine
1/2 onion, chopped
1/4 cup vegetable stock
Some lemon juice
Béchamel Sauce (Recipe no. 179)

Cut stalks into 1-1/2 in. pieces. Sauté in fat. Add stock, lemon juice and cook covered over low heat until tender, 1/2-3/4 hr. Add Béchamel Sauce, enriched with egg yolk and mix well together. Season with tarragon, bay, lemon, clove, onion, parsley and chives.

88. Mock Asparagus

3-4 pieces spinach beet stalks, prepared
1/2 tbsp. vegetable margarine
1/2 small onion, chopped
2 tbsp. milk or a little lemon juice
1/2 cup vegetable stock

Cut stalks into 4-in. pieces and sauté in the fat. Add lemon juice or milk. Add stock and cook over a small flame until tender, 1/2-3/4 hr. Season with tarragon, bay, cloves, chives. Arrange on a flat dish like asparagus. Serve with Béchamel or Tomato Sauce (recipes no. 179, 182).

Note: The stalks can also be sprinkled with grated cheese and hot butter.

89. Celery

3-4 celery stalks, prepared
1/2 tbsp. vegetable margarine
1/2 onion chopped
A little finely chopped apple
1/2 cup vegetable stock
2 tbsp. milk or a little lemon juice

Cut celery into 3-in. pieces. Melt fat, sauté celery briefly and cover. Add onion, apple, stock and milk. Cook for 1/2-3/4 hr. Season with celery leaves, vegetable fat.

90. Fennel

1 large or 2 small fennel
1/2 tbsp. vegetable fat
Some onion
1/2 cup vegetable stock
2 tbsp. milk or lemon juice
1/2 tbsp. flour
2-3 tbsp. milk (opt.)
Cheese (opt.)

Halve fennel, place in pan. Briefly sauté onion. Add fennel and sauté together with onion. Add stock, cook until tender. Very briefly, cook flour, milk and cheese and pour over the prepared fennel.

91. Swiss Chard

2-3 stalks Swiss chard
1/2 tbsp. vegetable margarine
Some lemon juice
1/2 cup vegetable stock

Clean and wash chard and cut stalks into 4-in. pieces.
Put in the pan, cover with melted margarine and lemon.
Cook until tender, 3/4-1 hr. Arrange on a plate, sprinkle
with cheese and melted butter. Season with lovage, clove.

92. Steamed Carrots

    1 tbsp. vegetable margarine or oil
    1/2 small onion
    3-4 carrots, sliced (or cut into strips)
    1/2 cup vegetable stock
    Pinch sugar

Brown onion in the fat. Add carrots, sugar and stock.
Cook for 1/2-3/4 hr. until tender. Season with parsley,
marjoram, thyme, or rosemary.

93. Creamed Carrots I

    1/4 tbsp. vegetable margarine
    3-4 carrots
    1/2 tbsp. vegetable margarine
    1/2 tbsp. flour
    1/2 cup milk
    1/2 cup water or vegetable stock

Melt 1/4 tbsp. margarine. Slice carrots finely and sauté
in the fat until they are nearly cooked. Melt 1/2 tbsp.
vegetable fat, stir flour into it. Gradually add milk and water,
or vegetable stock, to make a thin sauce. Add carrots. Cook
gently all together until carrots are done, about 1/2 hr.
Season with sugar browned in butter, sautéed onions, parsley, rosemary, marjoram, a piece of bay leaf, thyme,
tarragon.

94. Creamed Carrots, II

1 cup vegetable stock
3-4 carrots
1 tbsp. vegetable margarine
1 scant tbsp. flour
1/2 cup milk or juice from cooked carrots

Slice carrots and cook until soft in the vegetable stock.
Make a Béchamel Sauce with the ingredients given (Recipe
no. 179). Pour sauce over the cooked carrots. Season with
parsley, rosemary, marjoram, a little bay, thyme.

95. Peas and Carrots

1/4 tbsp. vegetable margarine
Some onion
4 oz. peas, shelled
1/2 cup vegetable stock
6 oz. carrots, peeled

Melt fat for the peas, sauté onion in it. Add peas, stock
and seasoning, and simmer until cooked. Melt fat for the
carrots, sauté onion in it. Add carrots, stock and seasoning
and simmer until cooked. Mix peas and carrots in one
saucepan or arrange alternately on a serving dish. Season
with sugar, browned in butter, parsley, chives, marjoram,
thyme, lovage.

96. Peas

1/2 tbsp. vegetable margarine
Onion
1/2 lb. shelled peas
1/2 cup vegetable stock
1/2 tbsp. sugar
1/2 oz. melted butter

Melt fat and sauté onion in it. Add peas, stock and simmer over a low flame until cooked soft, 20-40 min. according to quality. Season with sugar browned in butter, parsley, chives, marjoram, thyme, lovage. Serve with hot butter poured over the finished dish.

97. Peas, French Style

1/2 tbsp. vegetable margarine
1/2 onion
1/4 head Boston or Romaine lettuce (finely shredded)
5-7 oz. peas, shelled
1/2 cup vegetable stock
1/2 oz. fresh butter mixed with 1 tbsp. flour

Sauté onion in fat. Add vegetables and stock and simmer gently until peas are tender. Add a mixture of butter and flour to thicken liquid. Season with chives, parsley, marjoram, lovage.

98. Peas with Pearl Onions

1/2 tbsp. vegetable margarine
2-1/2 oz. pearl onions
1/2 lb. shelled peas
1/2 cup vegetable stock

Melt fat and sauté onion in it. Add peas, cover and simmer until cooked. Sprinkle chopped basil over the finished dish before serving. Season with parsley, chives, marjoram, thyme, lovage, fresh butter.

99. Steamed Chinese Peas

1/2 tbsp. vegetable margarine
1/2 onion, chopped
7 oz. Chinese peas, prepared
1/2 cup vegetable stock
Some parsley or lovage

Melt fat and sauté onion in it. Add sugar peas, salt and sauté all together. Add vegetable stock and herbs, cover and simmer 1/2-1 hr. (If preferred, the herbs can be sprinkled over the finished dish.) Season with chives, marjoram, thyme; add fresh or browned butter.

100. Green Beans

1/2 tbsp. vegetable margarine
1/2 onion, chopped
Some garlic
1/2 lb. beans
Savory, parsley
1/2 cup vegetable stock, or 1-2 tomatoes, diced

Melt fat and sauté onion and garlic in it. Add beans and sauté together. Add stock and herbs, cover and cook gently for 1 hr. In place of vegetable stock, diced tomatoes can be used, adding a little stock if too dry. Season with some caraway, marjoram, lovage.

101. Steamed Celeriac

1/2 tbsp. vegetable margarine
1/2 onion
1/2 celeriac, prepared
1/2 cup vegetable stock
2 tbsp. milk

Melt fat and sauté onion in it. Cut celeriac into thin small slices. Sauté with the onion. Add vegetable stock and cook until tender (1/2-3/4 hr.). Add milk to refine the flavor Season with lemon, marjoram, apple, nuts.

102. Celeriac with Béchamel Sauce

1 small celeriac
Other ingredients as in Recipe no. 101

Prepare as in Recipe no. 101. When finished mix with Béchamel Sauce, Recipe no. 179 and serve. Season with lemon, apple, marjoram, nuts.

103. Celeriac Slices with Béchamel Sauce

1 medium celeriac, cut into quarters
1/4 cup milk
2 cups water
Béchamel Sauce (no. 179)

Cook celeriac with milk and water until tender. Cut into 1/2-in. slices and arrange fanlike on a hot dish. Pour Béchamel Sauce over the slices; or add cheese, breadcrumbs and melted butter.

104. Braised Salsify

About 1 lb. prepared salsify
1/2 tbsp. vegetable fat
1/2 onion
1/4 cup milk
1/2 cup vegetable stock

Cut salsify into finger-length pieces. Braise quickly in fat. Add milk, onion, and vegetable stock. Cook over a low flame for 1 hr. Season with lemon, basil, celery leaves, bay leaf, yeast extract (parsley, onion, chives).

105. Red Beets

1-1/2 lb. beets
1/2 tbsp. vegetable margarine
1/2 onion, chopped
1/2 cup vegetable stock
Pinch sugar
1/4 bay leaf
1/2 tbsp. flour
2 tbsp. milk

Cut off beet root tips and leaves about 3/4-in. above roots, and wash beets carefully. Cook in salted water until tender (2-3 hrs.; 25 min. in a pressure cooker). Pour cold water over beetroots. Peel and cut into fine slices. Melt fat and sauté onion in it. Add beets and all other ingredients except the flour and milk, and mix well. Simmer for 1/4 hr. Blend flour with a little cold water and add to the mixture to thicken juices. Season with lemon, lovage, caraway, lemon balm, nutmeg, a hint of garlic, parsley.

106. Jerusalem Artichokes

1/2 lb. Jerusalem artichokes
1/2 tbsp. vegetable margarine
1/2 onion
2 tbsp. milk

Cook like Potatoes in their Jackets. (Recipe no. 141.) Peel and slice. Melt fat and sauté onion in it. Add Jerusalem artichokes and sauté together. Add milk and refine flavor. Season with basil.

107. Steamed Tomatoes

1 tbsp. oil
1/2 tbsp. vegetable margarine
1/2 onion
Sugar
4-5 tomatoes
A hint of garlic
Some cornstarch (opt.)

Melt fat and sauté onion in it. Cut up tomatoes and add to onion. Sauté gently. Add garlic and cook until tender. Thicken with cornstarch. Sprinkle liberally with chopped parsley or other herbs before serving. Season tomatoes with a little chopped parsley or other herbs such as rosemary, marjoram, basil, bay leaf, nutmeg, chives, dill, parsley.

108. Baked Tomatoes

2-3 tomatoes
1/2 oz. butter

Halve tomatoes and put in a baking dish. Put a dab of butter on each tomato and bake in a moderate oven.

If desired a few more tomatoes may be chopped finely (or put through a blender), brought to a boil with a little milk, and poured over the baked tomatoes. Season with parsley, sautéed onion.

109. Tomatoes with Cheese Slices

2 tomatoes
1 oz. cheese slice for each tomato

Halve tomatoes and put in a baking dish. Place a slice of cheese on each tomato. Bake in a moderate oven until the cheese is melted. Season with parsley.

110. Stuffed Tomatoes

2-3 tomatoes
3 tsp. rice
Butter or oil
Herbs
Some vegetable stock (if needed)

Cut tops off tomatoes. Remove and chop up pulp, mix with rice (1 tsp. per tomato), add herbs to taste and stuff the tomatoes. Top with dabs of butter and add stock. Bake in a moderate oven for about 30 min. Grated cheese may be sprinkled on top. Season with browned sugar, onion, garlic, rosemary, marjoram, thyme, basil, bay leaf, nutmeg, parsley, chives, dill.

111. Zucchini

1/2 tbsp. vegetable margarine
Onion, chopped
1 tbsp. oil
About 12 oz. (small) zucchini
2 oz. tomatoes
Pearl onions, chopped

Braise the onion. Cut the zucchini into cubes (for large zucchini, remove the seeds). Peel the tomatoes and cut into cubes. Braise the pearl onions and add at the end to the finished zucchini, or finish cooking the zucchini together with the tomato cubes.

If too much liquid forms, some corn starch can be stirred in for thickening. Season with garlic, rosemary, marjoram, thyme, basil, bay leaf, nutmeg, parsley, chives, dill.

112. Fried Squash or Zucchini

About 7 oz. zucchini or squash
Flour for coating
1 tbsp. oil or vegetable margarine

Cut zucchini into finger-length strips or into 1/2-in. slices. Coat with flour and fry immediately in oil or margarine.

113. French Fried Squash or Zucchini

These can be made exactly like French fried potatoes. Slice into hot oil or margarine and remove with a slotted spoon as soon as they are lightly browned.

114. Steamed Green or Yellow Peppers

(Best served as a side dish.)

5-7 oz. peppers
1 tbsp. oil
1/2 onion

Remove pith and seeds carefully. Slice peppers into strips and put into a saucepan with the oil and onion. Cover and steam gently for 1/2 hr. Season with garlic, rosemary, marjoram, thyme, basil, bay leaf, nutmeg, parsley.

115. Peppers Provencale

2 oz. green peppers
4 oz. squash or zucchini
2 oz. eggplant
1 tomato
1/2 onion
A little garlic
1 tbsp. oil
1 oz. potatoes

Halve peppers, remove pith and seeds and dice. Peel and dice squash and eggplant. Skin tomato and cut into large cubes. Chop onion and garlic and sauté in the oil. Add other diced vegetables and sauté together. Cut potatoes into 1/2-in. cubes, add to the other vegetables. Cook very slowly for 1 to 1-1/2 hrs. in a covered saucepan. If too much liquid forms, cook uncovered until it is reduced. Season with rosemary, marjoram, thyme, basil, bay, nutmeg, parsley.

116. Eggplant

7 oz. eggplant
Oil, for frying
1 tomato

Peel eggplant cut into slices and cook in oil until tender. Put into a baking dish. Slice tomato and put on top of eggplant. Sprinkle with cheese, grated or sliced, or bread crumbs. Dot with butter and bake in a medium oven for 1/2 hr.

117. Artichokes

1 artichoke
1 tbsp. lemon juice
3 cups water

Prepare artichokes by cutting off stems and removing tough outer leaves. Cut off tips of other leaves. Halve, cut out choke, wash well. Rub cut surfaces with lemon juice. Bring water to a boil, add artichokes and salt and cook until tender (3/4 hr. approx.). Drain, arrange on a hot dish covered with a napkin. Serve with Béchamel Sauce (Recipe no. 179) or Vinaigrette.

118. Asparagus

1/2 bunch asparagus
4 cups water

Wash the asparagus carefully without breaking and peel. Boil until tender for 20-30 min. in a long or wide pan. Take out with a slotted spoon and arrange on a hot dish covered with a napkin. Serve with grated cheese and melted margarine, Vinaigrette or lemon juice.

119. Corn On The Cob

1-2 ears of corn
4 cups water

Choose only ears with corn that is young and milky. Remove husks and silk. Boil until tender (10-20 min. according to freshness). Arrange on a hot dish covered with a napkin; serve with hot butter.

120. Cauliflower

1 small cauliflower
4 cups water

Cut off the cauliflower leaves and remove stalk close to the flowers. Cut into large pieces, peel stalk and keep tender leaves. Put into cold salt water for 1 hr. Rinse well. Cook until tender (20-30 min.); take out and drain well. Arrange on a hot deep dish. Serve with Béchamel Sauce, Recipe no 179; or with 1 tbsp. melted butter; or with tarragon butter and lemon; or with fresh butter, parsley, chives.

121. Brussels Sprouts

1/2 tbsp. vegetable margarine
7 oz. Brussels sprouts, cleaned
1/2 cup vegetable stock

Melt fat and sauté sprouts in it. Add stock and cook until tender (about 1/2 hr.). Before serving pour a little melted butter over them or Béchamel Sauce. Recipe no. 179. Season with nutmeg, basil.

Note: Large or tough sprouts should be blanched before they are cooked.

122. Steamed Cabbage

1/2 tbsp. vegetable margarine
1/2 onion chopped
8 oz. young cabbage
1/2 cup vegetable stock
Basil or lovage

Some yeast extract
Nutmeg
Caraway seeds

Melt fat and sauté onion in it. Cut the cabbage into 1/2-in. wide strips and sauté with the onion. Add stock gradually and simmer until tender, 1/2 hr. on a low flame. Add salt, herbs and spices to taste. Season with garlic, parsley.
Note: Blanch tough or old cabbage before cooking.

123. Chopped Cabbage

1/2 cabbage
5 cups water
1 tbsp. vegetable margarine
1/2 chopped onion
Garlic
1 scant tbsp. flour
1/2 cup vegetable stock or half milk, half vegetable stock
Yeast extract (opt.) or 1-2 tbsp. milk
Nutmeg

Cut cabbage into quarters. Cook in water until tender. Drain well and chop finely. Melt fat and sauté onion in it. Sprinkle flour over onion and sauté. Add stock and simmer for 1/4 hr. Add cabbage and bring to a boil again. Add yeast extract, nutmeg and salt. Season with caraway, parsley.

124. Savoy Cabbage

Prepare and cook as for Chopped Cabbage, Recipe no. 123.

125. Sour White Cabbage

1 tbsp. vegetable margarine or oil
1/2 onion
6 oz. white cabbage
1/2 tbsp. lemon juice
1/4 cup vegetable stock
1/4 cup apple juice
Caraway seeds

Melt fat and sauté onion in it. Shred cabbage and add to the onion. Add lemon juice, stock, apple juice and caraway. Cover and cook gently for 1 hr. Season with a little garlic, lovage, nutmeg, apple, tomato.

126. Red Cabbage

1 tbsp. vegetable margarine
1/2 onion, chopped
1/2 lb. red cabbage, shredded
1/2 tbsp. lemon juice
1/2 apple, thinly sliced
1/2 tbsp. rice
1/2 cup vegetable stock
1/4 cup grape or apple juice
1 apple, peeled, sliced
Butter

Melt fat and sauté onion in it. Add finely shredded raw cabbage, rice, lemon juice and sliced 1/2 apple and sauté all together. Add stock and fruit juice, cover pan and simmer until tended (1 to 1-1/2 hrs.). Peel the apple, remove core and cut into wedges; brush with butter and bake on a cooky sheet in the oven. Garnish red cabbage with the apples and dot with butter before serving.

127. Kohlrabi with Herbs

1 kohlrabi
1/2 tbsp. vegetable margarine
1/2 onion chopped
1/2 cup vegetable stock
1 tbsp. tender kohlrabi leaves, chopped
2 tbsp. milk (opt.)

Cut kohlrabi into quarters then slice finely. Melt fat and sauté the vegetables in it. Add stock, cover and cook gently for 1/2-1 hr. Add kohlrabi leaves and milk before serving. Add Béchamel Sauce, Recipe no. 179.

128. Steamed Leeks

7 oz. prepared leeks
1/2 tbsp. vegetable margarine
1/2 cup vegetable stock
2 tbsp. milk
Some grated cheese (opt.)

Cut leeks into 1-in. pieces. Melt fat and add leeks to the fat in layers. Pour vegetable stock over, cover and simmer until tender. Add cheese and milk just before serving.

129. Steamed Onions

1/2 tbsp. vegetable margarine
7 oz. pearl onions
Pinch of sugar
1/2 cup vegetable stock

Melt fat and sauté onions slowly in it; add sugar. Add stock and cook slowly for 3/4 hr. Garnish with peas or serve with Béchamel Sauce, Recipe no. 179.

130. Chestnuts as a Vegetable

8 oz. chestnuts
1/2 tbsp. vegetable margarine
1/2 tbsp. sugar
1/2 cup vegetable stock
2 tbsp. milk
2 tbsp. fresh butter

Cut two slits with a sharp knife in the form of a diagonal cross on the flat side of the chestnut shells. Place on a baking sheet in a hot oven until they split open; peel. Melt fat, add sugar and brown it. Add vegetable stock, chestnuts. Cook for 1/2 hr. until liquid has evaporated. Add butter to the chestnuts before serving.

Note: If preferred, omit the sugar and sauté the chestnuts with chopped onion. Add vegetable stock and cook. Serve garnished with strips of fried onion.

131. Purée of Split Peas

4-6 oz. split peas, yellow or green
(soaked overnight)
1 small potato
1/2 cup milk
Vegetable stock if required
1 tomato diced
1/2 onion
1/2 tbsp. vegetable margarine
1 tbsp. croutons
1-1/2 tbsp. butter

Cook peas and potato in the water used for soaking, until quite tender, drain well and strain. Add milk to make a thick purée; add stock if required; keep warm over boiling water. Sauté tomatoes and onion in margarine and use

to garnish. Fry bread cubes in remaining margarine or
butter and serve with finished dish.

132. Lentils

6 oz. lentils (soaked overnight)
7 oz. vegetable stock
1 onion with 3-4 cloves pressed into it
1/2 tbsp. vegetable margarine
1/2 onion chopped
1/2 tbsp. flour
1/2 tbsp. lemon juice, or
    2 tbsp. milk

Drain soaked lentils well. Add vegetable stock, and
onion with cloves, to the lentils. Cook until tender. Melt
margarine and sauté onion in it. Sprinkle flour over lentils
and add sautéed onion. Add lemon juice or milk.

133. Mixed Vegetables

1 tbsp. margarine
1/2 onion
2 oz. celeriac
2 oz. carrots
1/2 cup vegetable stock
2 oz. cauliflower
1/2 cup milk and water, mixed
2 oz. green peas or beans
1/2 cup vegetable stock

Sauté onion. Dice celeriac and carrots and sauté with the
onion. Add 1/2 cup stock and cook until tender. Cook
peas or beans in remaining stock. Cook cauliflower in milk
and water until tender. Mix all cooked vegetables together.

COOKED VEGETABLE SALADS

Carrots, celery roots, beets, beans, cauliflower, Chinese artichokes are particularly suitable for these salads.

The vegetable should be cooked until tender in vegetable stock or water and then cut into small segments (slices, strips, rosettes). Dress with a salad dressing or mayonnaise. Cauliflower can also be garnished with a Remoulade Sauce (Recipe no. 190). Flavor with chopped herbs and onions.

134. Potato Salad

    8 oz. potatoes
    1/4 cup vegetable stock, hot
    1 tbsp. oil
    1 tbsp. lemon juice
    1/2 tbsp. onion, chopped

Boil potatoes, peel and slice while they are still hot. Cover with hot vegetable stock, and let stand for a short time. Mix oil and lemon juice and pour over potatoes. Add onions. Season with borage, parsley, dill, lemon balm, chives, marjoram.

135. Potato Salad With Cucumbers

    1 large potato
    1/4 cucumber
    1/2 tbsp. oil
    1/2 tbsp. lemon juice

Prepare potatoes as for Potato Salad (Recipe no. 134). Grate cucumber coarsely. Beat oil, lemon juice together and mix with potato salad. Season with onion, borage, dill, chives. Rub salad bowl with garlic.

136. Mixed Salad

Choose 3-4 different varieties of vegetable such as carrots, celeriac, Chinese artichokes, zucchini, beetroot, potatoes, beans.

Take the cooked vegetables and dice or slice them. Mix with French Dressing (Recipe no. 7). Season with yeast extract, chives, parsley, dill, marjoram, thyme.

137. Nicoise Salad

1 cooked potato
1 small tomato
Radishes
A few slices of cucumber
1 tbsp. oil
1/2 tbsp. lemon juice
A few Boston lettuce leaves

Slice vegetables. Prepare French Dressing (Recipe no. 7) and mix with vegetables. Add lettuce leaves to the salad shortly before serving. Season with chives or dill, borage, parsley, lemon balm.

Note: Can also be made with soy mayonnaise (Recipe no. 8).

138. Rice Salad

2 oz. rice
7 oz. water
1 tbsp. oil
1/2 tbsp. lemon juice
1/2 tbsp. onion, chopped
1/2 tomato, diced small

Cook rice in the water until soft. Rinse well under water. Let stand until cold. Mix oil and lemon juice together thoroughly and add to rice. Mix diced tomatoes and onion and add to the other ingredients. Arrange finished salad on lettuce leaves or serve in shells. Season with chives, parsley and basil.

139. Celeriac Salad with Soy Mayonnaise

1/2 small celeriac, raw
1/2-1 tbsp. lemon juice
2 walnuts, roughly chopped or 1/4 apple, grated (opt.)
1 tbsp. mayonnaise (no. 8)

Shred celeriac very finely and mix with lemon juice. Chop walnuts, grate apple, and add to celeriac. Mix carefully with Mayonnaise Dressing (Recipe no. 8).

140. Vegetable Aspic

1 cup vegetable stock
1/2 heaping tsp. Agar-Agar*
A few drops of lemon juice
Yeast extract

---

* Agar-Agar is a vegetable gelatin made from seaweed. It can be used instead of gelatin for vegetables, desserts, sauces, puddings, etc., and is obtainable in powdered form at health food stores.

Egg slices
Diced tomato
Diced cucumber
Diced cauliflower florets
Cooked peas
Cooked beans

Dissolve the Agar-Agar in lukewarm stock, heat slowly, making sure it is completely dissolved. Add lemon juice and yeast extract to season. Pour a little aspic into individual molds or bowl, previously rinsed out in cold water. Chill. Top with egg and some of the vegetables, pour in a little more aspic and again leave to set. Continue in this manner adding vegetables and aspic alternately until the dish is full. When the aspic has set, turn out and use to garnish salad dishes.

POTATO DISHES

141. Potatoes in Their Jackets

Yellow or red potatoes are especially good done this way.

3-4 small potatoes
Water

Scrub the potatoes and wash well. Use a perforated insert or a wire basket within a saucepan. Fill with water to bottom of insert or basket. Add potatoes, cover and cook 30-40 min. Alternatively, use a pressure cooker.

142. Baked Potatoes

3-4 potatoes
1 tbsp. oil
Butter

Scrub the potatoes and wash well. Score skin on upper side three or four times, brush with oil. Bake on a greased baking sheet 30-40 min. in a moderate oven. Put a dab of butter on each potato before serving.

143. Potatoes with Cottage Cheese

3-4 small potatoes
1 tbsp. oil
1-2 tbsp. milk
2 oz. low-fat cottage cheese
Chives, or caraway, or marjoram

Score once across upper side of potatoes, bake in moderate oven 30-40 min. Mix cheese with milk, add herbs to taste. Put into a pastry bag and pipe over the slit in the baked potatoes. This mixture can also be used for baked potatoes.

144. Caraway Potatoes

2-3 medium-sized potatoes (long, narrow)
1 tsp. caraway seeds

Brush the potatoes and wash well. Halve potatoes across narrow side. Dip cut side of the potatoes into the caraway seeds. Place on a baking sheet, cut surface down; brush with oil. Bake in a moderate oven for 3/4 hr.

145. Potatoes in Vegetable Stock

Cubed celery and carrots are also cooked in the broth.

1/2 lb. potatoes
1/2-1 cup vegetable stock
1/2 oz. vegetable margarine

Wash potatoes, peel and cut into halves or pieces. Cook until tender in stock. Add margarine to the cooked potatoes. Season with lovage, some thyme, bay leaf, onion peel.

146. Parsley Potatoes

1/2 lb. potatoes
A little water
1 tbsp. fresh butter
1 tbsp. parsley, chopped

Wash and peel potatoes, cut into four lengthwise. Steam potatoes in a wire basket or steamer. Melt butter and mix with parsley, add to potatoes, serve.

147. Creamed Potatoes

7 oz. potatoes
1/2 tbsp. vegetable margarine
1/2 cup vegetable stock
1/4 cup milk
Parsley

Wash and peel potatoes, cut into slices. Melt fat, sauté potatoes lightly in it. Add stock, and cook slowly until tender. Add milk just before serving and sprinkle with parsley.

148. Potatoes with Tomatoes

1/2 tbsp. vegetable margarine
1/2 small onion
7 oz. potatoes
1/2 cup vegetable stock
1 small tomato
1 tbsp. milk

Melt fat, sauté onion in it. Add peeled, sliced potatoes, vegetable stock and salt, and cook gently. Skin tomato, slice and add to potatoes just before they are completely cooked. Add milk just before serving. Season with marjoram or rosemary or thyme, possibly nutmeg.

149. Potato Snow

4 potatoes
Water
Vegetable margarine

Wash and peel potatoes, cut into small pieces. Steam or boil in a little water, until cooked. Force through a sieve or colander on to a warm dish. Season with thinly sliced tomatoes or sautéed onion rings. Pour melted vegetable margarine over finished dish.

150. Mashed Potatoes

4 potatoes
Water
1/2 oz. butter
1/2 cup milk
Nutmeg

Peel potatoes, cut into small pieces. Steam or boil in a little water until tender. Melt butter and heat with the milk in a second saucepan. Force hot, cooked potatoes through a sieve or colander (or mash with a wooden spoon) into this saucepan. Beat all together until fluffy. Arrange on a hot dish; make patterns with a knife, dipped in hot water. Season with finely chopped marjoram, sautéed onion rings, garlic, grated and dried tomatoes, finely chopped caraway.

151. Potato Balls

4 potatoes
Water
1/2 cup milk
1/2 oz. butter
Nutmeg
1/2 oz. butter, melted

Prepare mashed potatoes (Recipe no. 150). Mix with milk. Dip small ladle into hot oil. Scoop out balls of potato and place on a hot dish. Garnish with melted butter (1/2 oz.). Season with nutmeg.

152. Browned Potatoes

2 small potatoes
Water
1/2 cup vegetable stock
1/2 tbsp. vegetable margarine (melted)
2-3 tbsp. milk

Peel potatoes, cut in half and parboil in a little water. Put in an oven-proof pan with the cut surfaces down. Pour vegetable stock and the melted fat over potatoes and braise in moderate oven until the vegetable stock has been absorbed. Pour milk over and continue roasting until the cut surfaces brown. Arrange on a hot dish with cut sides up, sprinkle with chopped parsley. Season with nutmeg, thyme, small bay leaf, small clove.

153. Hash Browns

4 potatoes, cooked the day before in their skins and allowed to cool
1 tbsp. vegetable margarine

Peel potatoes, cut into thin slices. Heat fat in a frying pan, add potatoes. Cover and brown potatoes, turning occasionally. Uncover at the last, to insure crispness. Using a spatula, form into a thick pancake, allow light brown crust to form on underside. Carefully turn over onto a hot dish. Season with parsley, chives.

Note: If liked, sauté chopped onion in butter and add to the potatoes before the last browning.

154. Lyons Potatoes

1/2 tbsp. margarine
1/2 tbsp. oil
3 small potatoes, peeled
1 small onion, sliced in strips

Heat fat and oil in a frying pan. Peel potatoes, cut into slices. Cook in the hot fat until half done. Add onions, and finish cooking.

155. Potato Sticks

3 large potatoes
1/2 tbsp. oil

Peel raw potatoes and cut into small sticks. Dry in a cloth. Heat oil, add potatoes. Cover with a lid and steam for a short time. Remove lid and allow to brown for about 1/2 hr. Season with some nutmeg and rosemary.

156. French Fried Potatoes

3 potatoes, peeled
Vegetable margarine or oil

Cut potatoes into thin French fries, dry at once in a cloth. Heat fat or oil. Deep-fry potatoes a few at a time for 5-10 min. Take out with perforated spoon, drain on a rack or grease-proof paper, or use a deep-fat fryer. Shortly before serving heat up oil again and fry potatoes quickly so that they are crisp outside but remain soft inside. Drain again, and serve immediately. Garnish with some sprigs of parsley briefly dipped in the vegetable oil.

157. Potato Chips

1 large potato, peeled
Oil or vegetable margarine

Slice the potato thinly straight into the smoking fat. Fry until golden. Drain and serve immediately.

158. Potato Cakes with Spinach

1 large potato
1/2 cup vegetable stock
1/4 lb. spinach
1 tbsp. cheese (grated)
Butter

Peel potato and cut lengthwise into approx. 1/2-in. slices. Cook potato carefully until tender, place slices on a greased baking sheet. Cook the spinach (as in Recipe no. 83) and heap onto potato slices. Sprinkle on grated cheese. Put dabs of butter on top. Bake in moderate oven for a few minutes. Season with sautéed onion, some garlic, parsley, chives, possibly mint or some sage and nutmeg.

159. Potatoes with Savoy Cabbage

1/2 tbsp. vegetable margarine
1 tbsp. chopped onion
4 oz. Savoy cabbage, cut up
2 small potatoes, diced
Melted butter

Melt fat, sauté onion in it. Add chopped cabbage and sauté. Add diced potatoes and sauté all together. Add stock, cover, and cook for 1/2-3/4 hr. Melt butter and pour over finished vegetables. Season with some finely chopped caraway, marjoram, nutmeg, or basil.

GRAIN DISHES

160. Japanese Rice

1/2 tbsp. vegetable margarine
3 oz. rice*
3/4-1 cup vegetable bouillon or celery water
1 small onion, peeled and stuck with a bay leaf and
    clove
1/2 oz. butter

---

* We prefer to use brown rice for all but dessert dishes. Follow cooking time on the package.

Melt fat, add rice and sauté. Add water and onion, cover and cook for about 15 min. Cool rice, which should be separate and grainy. Heat butter, add cooked rice and sauté until really hot. Put dabs of butter on the finished rice before serving.

161. Risotto

1/2 tbsp. vegetable margarine
1 tbsp. chopped onion
3 oz. brown rice
7 oz. vegetable stock or water
1/2 oz. fresh butter

Sauté rice and onion in margarine. Then cook in stock for 30-40 min. Mix in margarine using a fork. Season with dried mushrooms, chopped, fresh herbs to taste, rosemary.

162. Saffron Rice

Prepare as for Risotto (Recipe no. 161), but add a pinch of saffron power dissolved in bouillon to the stock. Season with dried mushrooms, chopped fresh herbs according to taste, rosemary.

163. Créole Rice

1/2 tbsp. vegetable margarine
1 tbsp. onion, chopped
3 oz. brown rice
7 oz. water or stock

Melt vegetable fat, sauté onion and rice in it until transparent. Add heated stock, cook 30-40 min. Season with yeast extract, bay leaf, clove, possibly nutmeg.

164. Créole Rice with Vegetables

1/2 tbsp. vegetable margarine
2 tbsp. vegetables, very finely diced (leek, celery, carrots)
3 oz. brown rice
7 oz. vegetable stock

Sauté vegetables and rice in fat. Add hot stock and cook for 30-40 min. Season with freshly chopped herbs according to taste, bay leaf, cloves, perhaps some nutmeg.

165. Rice with Tomatoes

3 oz. brown rice
1/2 tbsp. vegetable margarine
Some garlic
1 tbsp. onion, chopped
1/2 cup vegetable stock
1 large tomato
1/2 oz. butter

Sauté onion and garlic. Add rice, braise until shiny. Peel the tomato, cube and add. Add stock, cook for 30-40 min. Finally, mix in butter. Season with rosemary, marjoram, clove, bay leaf, possibly basil or nutmeg. Mix in a little sugar if tomatoes and onions are used.

166. Risotto with Peppers

1 tbsp. oil
1 tbsp. onion, chopped
1/2 pepper
2 oz. brown rice
1/2 cup vegetable stock

Cut pepper in half, remove seeds and pith and cut into strips. Heat oil and sauté onion and peppers in it. Add rice and sauté all together. Add stock and cook on the top of the stove or in the oven for 45 min. Season with rosemary, marjoram, clove, bay leaf, possibly basil, nutmeg.

Note: If the pepper is bitter, score across the thick part and soak in cold water for 1 hr. before cooking.

167. Risotto with Zucchini

1 tbsp. onion, chopped
1/2 lb. zucchini (small)
1/2 tbsp. vegetable margarine
Vegetable stock or water
3 oz. brown rice
3/4 cup water or vegetable stock
1/2 oz. fresh butter

Sauté the onion. Dice zucchini and sauté together for 10 min. Add rice and stock gradually until the mixture forms a risotto. Mix in butter. Season with yeast extract and freshly chopped dill.

168. Risotto with Peas

1/2 tbsp. vegetable margarine or oil
Some onion, chopped
6 oz. shelled peas
Some sugar
1/4 cup vegetable stock
3 oz. brown rice
3/4-1 cups water
1/2 oz. butter

Melt fat and sauté chopped onion in it until golden brown. Add peas, and sauté with onion. Add 1/4 cup

vegetable stock and cook until tender. Prepare a risotto
with the next 4 ingredients. When cooked, add cooked
peas to it. Add butter to the finished dish. Season with
chopped parsley, or clove.

169. Rice with Spinach

1/2 tbsp. margarine or oil
Some onion, chopped
4 oz. spinach, cut coarsely
3 oz brown rice
7 oz. vegetable stock or water
1/2 oz. fresh butter

Sauté onion, spinach, rice. Add stock, cook together for
30-40 min. Mix in butter. Season with nutmeg and mint.

170. Pilaff with Tomatoes

1/2 tbsp. margarine or oil
2 tbsp. vegetables, chopped very finely
   (leek, celery, carrots)
3 oz. brown rice
3/4 cup vegetable stock
2 small tomatoes, sliced
1/2 oz. butter

Sauté vegetables and rice. Heat stock, add to vegetables
and rice. Cook for 30-40 min. Put alternate layers of rice
and tomatoes in a well-greased baking dish. Sprinkle pieces
of butter over the dish and bake for 10 min. Season with
parsley, lovage, braised onions.

171. Farina Pudding

2 oz. farina
1-1/4 cups milk
7 oz. water
1 tbsp. sugar
1/2 oz. vegetable margarine

Combine milk and water. Stir farina into hot liquid. Cook for 15-20 min. Pour melted fat over the prepared dish. Season with sugar and cinnamon.

172. Polenta

1/2 tbsp. oil
2 oz. yellow cornmeal
1-1/4 cups water
Nutmeg
1/2 tbsp. vegetable margarine
1 tbsp. grated cheese

Coat heavy pan with the oil. Bring water to the boil in the same saucepan. Stir cornmeal, and nutmeg into the boiling water and cook over a low flame for 5 min., stirring continuously. Then cook slowly, covered, for 1-2 hours. Mix in fat with a fork.

Note: Sautéed onion slices and fresh margarine can be spread over the Polenta, if desired.

173. Millotto

1/2 tbsp. vegetable margarine or oil
1 tbsp. onion, chopped
2 oz. millet
3/4 cup vegetable stock, hot
1 tbsp. cheese
1/2 oz. butter
1/2 onion, cut into rings

Sauté chopped onion and rice in oil until it becomes transparent. Cook millet in stock for 20 min. Sprinkle cheese and sautéed onion rings over cooked dish.

174. Millotto with Vegetables

1/2 tbsp. vegetable margarine or oil
1 tbsp. onion, chopped
1 tbsp. diced vegetables (leek, celery, carrots, or
    carrots and peas)
1-1/2 oz. millet
3/4 cup vegetable stock
1 tbsp. cheese
1/2 oz. fresh butter

Sauté vegetables, millet and onion. Add stock and cook for 20 min. Sprinkle cheese and butter over the prepared dish. Season with rosemary and yeast extract.

175. Porridge

2 tbsp. cracked wheat, oats or rye
3 tbsp. water

Soak cereals for 12 hrs. Add 2-3 tbsp. water to the soaked cereals, and cook for 10 min. in a saucepan or for 1/2 hr. in a double boiler.

176. Spinach Noodles

(Homemade for 4 persons.)

> 1-3/4 cups flour (1/2 whole-wheat)
> 4 oz. raw spinach, chopped
> 2 eggs
> 1 tbsp. water
> 1 tbsp. oil

Sift flour, make a well in the center. Add other ingredients and mix into a smooth dough. Let stand for 1/2 hr. Using only half the dough, roll it out paper thin and set aside; repeat for the other half. After about 1 hr. roll up each sheet and cut in fine strips. The noodles are now ready to be cooked. Season with sautéed onion.

177. Soya Gnocchi

> 1/2 cup whole-wheat flour
> 1-1/2 oz. soy flour
> 1/2 cup water, salt
> 1 tbsp. grated cheese (opt.)

Make a well in the center of the flour, add eggs and water, beat well until bubbles form. Put aside for at least 1 hr. Bring salted water to the boil. Force batter, a small portion at a time, through a sieve with a large perforation into the boiling water. Simmer until gnocchi rise to the surface. Take out with a slotted spoon and arrange on dish. Sprinkle with grated cheese. Season with sliced onion sautéed in vegetable margarine, or with plain melted fat; chives, parsley or tomatoes. Gnocchi can also be cooked in vegetable stock and arrange immediately on a hot dish.

178. Spinach or Tomato Gnocchi

5 oz. flour (1/3 whole-wheat)
1-1/2 oz. soy flour
1/2 cup milk and water, mixed
1 handful chopped raw spinach or 1 tsp. tomato
   purée
4 cups water

Prepare a smooth batter of the first 4 ingredients and put aside for 1 hr. Cook as in Recipe no. 177. Season with sliced onion sautéed in vegetable fat, or with oil or melted fat, chives or tomatoes.

OPEN-FACE SANDWICHES

Open-face sandwiches (canapés) are easily digestible and generally enjoyed, either as an hors d'oeuvre or light supper dish in summer. They are excellent also for teas, buffets and cocktail parties. Sandwiches or small rolls can also be taken on picnics or for packed lunches. The fillings can be varied almost indefinitely, the fresher and more colorful and attractive the slices look, the more appetizing they will prove.

Whole-wheat bread should be at least one day old so that it may be cut into really thin slices.

BASIC SPREADS:

Vegetable margarine or 1 oz. cottage cheese
1 tsp. butter, whipped
Yeast extract mixed with 2 tbsp. milk
Chives, herbs or caraway, or herb butter with dill
   or borage and some milk mixed in

Garnishes: The open sandwiches can be decorated with, raw carrot or celery, or with tomatoes, cucumber, radishes, cress, onion rings, olives, parsley, chives, etc.

SAUCES

179. Béchamel Sauce

1/2 tbsp. vegetable margarine
1 tbsp. flour
1/4 cup milk
1/4 cup vegetable stock or water
Nutmeg

Melt fat, add flour and sauté. Add the liquid slowly, stirring all the time. Cook for 20 min.

180. Herb Sauce

Make Béchamel Sauce as in Recipe no. 179. Season with with chervil, basil, tarragon, parsley, lovage, etc.

181. Tomato Sauce I

1/2 tbsp. vegetable margarine or oil
1 tbsp. onion
Some garlic
2 tbsp. diced carrots, celery and leek
2 small tomatoes
Some flour
3/4 cup vegetable stock or water
A little hot butter
Pinch of sugar

Cut up vegetables. Melt fat and sauté onions and garlic in it. Add vegetables and sauté in the fat. Cut up tomatoes and add. Cook slowly until juices have been reduced. Sprinkle flour over vegetables. Add stock or water and cook for 1/2 hr. Strain through a sieve. Add butter and sugar to enrich the flavor. Season with bay leaf, rosemary, thyme.

182. Tomato Sauce II

3 tomatoes
1 tbsp. butter

Cut tomatoes in pieces, cook till tender with salt and herbs. Strain. Add butter to improve flavor. Season with chives, basil.

183. Tomato Sauce III

1 tbsp. vegetable margarine or oil
1/2 small onion, chopped
2 tomatoes

Melt fat and sauté onion in it. Peel and dice tomatoes and add to the onion with salt and herbs. Cook till tender. Season with thyme, lemon juice, sugar.

184. Onion Sauce

1/2 tbsp. vegetable margarine or oil
1 small onion, cut in strips
1 tbsp. flour
1/2 cup vegetable stock
Some butter

Melt fat and sauté onion till golden brown. Mix in flour and cook till golden brown. Add stock and cook for 20 min. Strain, if desired. Stir in butter to enrich flavor. Season with nutmeg, yeast extract.

185. Horseradish Sauce

Béchamel Sauce, Recipe no. 179
1/2 oz. fresh horseradish

Prepare Béchamel Sauce, Recipe no. 179. Grate horseradish into the sauce. Cook for 5 min.

186. Brown Sauce

1/2 tbsp. vegetable margarine or oil
1 tbsp. flour
1/2 cup vegetable stock
2 tbsp. milk (opt.)

Melt fat, stir in flour and cook till chestnut brown. Take off the fire, add stock and cook for 20 min. Stir in milk, if desired. Season with ground cloves, lemon juice, nutmeg.

187. Mushroom Sauce

1/2 tbsp. vegetable margarine or oil
1 tbsp. onion, chopped
4 oz. fresh mushrooms
1/2 tbsp. flour
1/2 cup vegetable stock
Some lemon juice
2 tbsp. milk

Melt fat and sauté onion in it. Add mushrooms, thinly sliced. Sauté together, cover and cook for 1/4 hr. Sprinkle flour over. Add stock and lemon juice and cook for 10 min. Add milk to enrich the flavor of the sauce. Season with nutmeg, parsley, yeast extract.

188. Green Pepper Sauce

1/2 tbsp. vegetable margarine or oil
1 tbsp. onion, chopped
1 tbsp. green pepper, sliced finely
1 tbsp. flour
1/2 cup vegetable stock
2 tbsp. milk (opt.)

Melt fat, sauté onion and green pepper in it. Sprinkle flour over. Add stock, salt and bay leaf and cook for 20 min. Add milk to enrich sauce. Season with bay leaf.

189. Soy Mayonnaise

(Without animal protein, for 4 persons.)

2 level tbsp. soy flour
6 tbsp. water
1/2 cup oil
4 tbsp. lemon juice

Blend flour and water, and whisk until smooth. Add oil and lemon juice drop by drop, whisking all the time. Add herbs to season as above.

190. Rémoulade Sauce

Prepare as Soy Mayonnaise in Recipe no. 189. Add 2 tbsp. diced tomatoes to garnish. Season as above.

DESSERTS

These recipes are for 4 persons.

191. Sugar Syrup

2-4 oz. sugar (raw or granulated)
1-1/2 cups water or 3/4 cup water, and 3/4 cup grape juice
Approx. 2 lbs. apricots or peaches, damsons, plums, greengages

Dissolve sugar in water and bring to the boil. Halve fruit and remove stones. Cook briefly in the syrup; cool. Arrange attractively in a dish.

192. Strawberries with Lemon Juice

1-1/2 lb. hulled strawberries (approx. 2 pt.)
1 lemon
2-3 tbsp. sugar

Halve large strawberries, add sugar and lemon juice.

193. Fruit Salad

3-1/2 oz. sugar (raw or granulated)
1/2 cup water
1/2-1 cup grape juice or apple juice
Approx. 1-1/2 lbs. apricots or peaches, melon,
    apples, pears (soft type), red cherries (pitted),
    or any variety of berry

Prepare a selection of fruit according to the season. Dissolve sugar in the water, then bring to the boil. Add fruit juices. Slice fruit finely and add to the cooled syrup.

194. Stuffed Melon

2 small melons
Fruit Salad, Recipe no. 193

Halve melons and remove seeds. Fill with the fruit salad.

195. Fruit Jello

1-1/2 cups water or grape juice
3 oz. sugar
1 tbsp. Agar-Agar*
3 cups juice (orange, berries)

Whisk water or grape juice with sugar and heat slowly with Agar-Agar until completely dissolved. Mix in fresh fruit juice and pour at once into glasses or small dishes to set.

---

* See note for recipe no. 140.

196. Apple Sauce

2 lbs. apples
1 cup water or apple juice
3-4 oz. raw sugar
Cinnamon or lemon peel

Peel and core apples and cut into pieces. Add water and bring to a boil. Mix in sugar, cinnamon. Cook until tender. As a refinement, a tablespoon of roasted sugar may be sprinkled over the sauce.

197. Apple Compote

2 lbs. apples
1 to 1-1/2 cups water or apple juice
4 oz. sugar
Peel of 1 lemon, grated, or some cinnamon

Peel and core the apples and cut into slices. Bring the liquid to a boil. Add sugar, lemon peel and apples and cook until tender.

198. Apple Halves

2 lbs. apples
2 cups water or apple juice
5-1/2 oz. sugar
1/4 stick cinnamon
Quince, raspberry or red currant jelly

Peel apples, cut in half, and remove cores. Bring liquid to the boil, flavor with sugar and cinnamon, add the apples, a portion at a time, and cook until tender. Remove with slotted spoon, put on a dish, cut surfaces. Fill with a dab of jelly.

199. Blueberry Sweet

2 lbs. blueberries
7 oz. raw or granulated sugar
3/4 cup water
1 tbsp. flour
2 tbsp. water
1 oz. bread cubes (salt-free bread)
1 oz. vegetable margarine

Wash fruit. Cook 5-10 min. in water with sugar. Blend flour with some water, add to blueberries with the rest of the water and bring to the boil. Put into serving dish. Sauté bread cubes in fat and use as a garnish.

200. Stewed Rhubarb

2 lbs. rhubarb
2-7 oz. raw or granulated sugar
1/2 cup water
1/2 tbsp. cornstarch

Wash rhubarb, cut into small pieces. Cook in water, with sugar, until tender. Remove with slotted spoon and put into a serving dish. Boil juice to thicken, or mix 1/2 tbsp. cornstarch with water, add to the juice and bring to the boil. Pour over rhubarb.

201. Strawberry Cup

1 lb. strawberries
4 oz. sugar

Mix the ingredients together or first put the berries through a sieve or blender then add sugar.

Note: Other fruit may be prepared in the same manner.

202. Vanilla Cup

1 lb. fruit
1 cup water
2-3 tbsp. sugar
1/2 serving Vanilla Cream (Recipe no. 207)

Prepare a compote of fruit, sugar and water. Pour Vanilla Cream over prepared dish.

203. Junket with Fruit

3 cups milk
1-2 tbsp. sugar, with vanilla or grate lemon peel
1/2 junket tablet
1 tbsp. water
Fresh, sugared berries

Heat the milk and flavored sugar to about 98°F. Crush the junket tablet, dissolve it in water, add to the hot milk. Stir well. Pour into glasses or bowls immediately. When junket has set, refrigerate. Shortly before serving the junket add fresh, ripe berries.

204. Stuffed Apples

4 large or 8 small apples
4 tbsp. grated filberts
2 tbsp. currants
3 tbsp. sugar
4 tbsp. milk
Gratel peel of 1 lemon
1/2 oz. vegetable margarine
1 tbsp. sugar
1/2-3/4 cup apple juice

Wipe apples, core and make an incision round the apple skin. Mix nuts, currants, milk, sugar and lemon. Put apples into a baking dish and fill centers with mixture. Top with dabs of butter, sprinkle with sugar. Pour juice to a depth of about 1/2 in., bake 20-30 min.

205. Caramel Pears

2 lbs. pears
7 oz. sugar
2-3 cups boiling water
1/2 tsp. cornstarch
1/4 cup milk

Peel pears, cut in half and remove cores. Brown sugar over low heat then cook gently in water until golden brown. Add pears and cook until tender. Lift out fruit with slotted spoon and arrange in a glass dish; about 2 cups liquid should remain. Mix cornstarch with milk, add to the boiling juice, bring again to the boil. Pour hot sauce over pears.

206. Apple Hedgehog with Vanilla Cream

2 lbs. apples (prepared as in no. 198)
1-1/4 cups milk
1/2 vanilla bean
1-2 tbsp. sugar
1 tsp. cornstarch
1 egg (when allowed)
1-1/2 oz. almonds

Prepare apples as in Apple Halves, Recipe no. 198. From the next 5 ingredients prepare Vanilla Cream, Recipe no. 207. Cut almonds into thin slivers and lightly roast in oven. Mound apple halves, cut surfaces down, on a flat dish; spike with almond silvers to represent porcupine quills. Cover with Vanilla Cream.

207. Vanilla Cream

(If egg is allowed.)

3 cups milk
1 vanilla bean
1 tbsp. cornstarch
3 tbsp. milk
3 eggs
2-4 oz. sugar

Bring milk and vanilla to the boil. Mix cornstarch with cold milk, add to the hot milk, and bring again to the boil. Whisk sugar and eggs. Stir some hot liquid into the eggs, mixing well. Return whisked eggs to the same pan and stir until almost boiling again.

208. Strawberry or Raspberry Cream

11 oz. berries
1 cup milk
1/2 vanilla bean
1 tsp. cornstarch
1 tbsp. milk
1 egg
2-3 tbsp. sugar

Mix berries in blender or pass through a sieve. Prepare remaining ingredients as for Vanilla Cream (Recipe no. 207). Allow to cool and mix with the berries.

209. Apple Cream

1 cup milk
1/2 vanilla bean
1 tsp. cornstarch
1 tbsp. milk
1 egg
1 tbsp. sugar
14 oz. apples
1/4 cup water or apple juice
Grated lemon peel

Prepare cream as for Vanilla Cream (Recipe no. 207). Prepare a thick Apple Sauce (Recipe no. 196) using the apples, water, peel and sugar. Mix with the cream.

210. Rhubarb Cream

1 lb. rhubarb
3 to 3-1/2 oz. sugar
1 cup milk

1/2 vanilla bean
1 tsp. cornstarch
1 tbsp. milk
1 egg
1 tbsp. sugar

Wash rhubarb and dice. Cook until tender, with sugar. Put through blender or force through sieve. Prepare Vanilla Cream, Recipe no. 207 and cool. Mix with rhubarb, sprinkle with 1 tbsp. sugar.

211. Apricot Cream

Prepare as for Rhubarb Cream (Recipe no. 210) substituting apricots for rhubarb and adding 1 tsp. lemon juice.

212. Orange Cream

Prepare as for Lemon Cream, Recipe no. 214.

213. Uncooked Orange Cream

1 piece orange peel
1/2 cup water
1 scant tsp. powdered Agar-Agar
3/4 cup orange juice
1 tsp. lemon juice
5-6 tbsp. sugar
2 eggs

Whisk peel, water and Agar-Agar together. Heat gently until the Agar-Agar is completely dissolved. Stir in juices. Beat egg together with sugar, add to fruit cream.

214. Lemon Cream

3 cups milk
1-2 lemons
1 tbsp. cornstarch
3 tbsp. milk
3 eggs
3-1/2–5-1/2 oz. sugar

Peel lemons very thinly, and squeeze juice. Bring peel*
to the boil in the milk. Mix cornstarch with cold milk. Add
to boiling peel and milk, and bring again to the boil. Whisk
eggs and sugar, add a little of the boiling mixture, stir well.
Pour back into the saucepan, stirring constantly and bring
again to near boiling point. Cool, then strain. Add a few
spoonfuls lemon juice.

215. Uncooked Lemon Cream

1 piece lemon peel**
3/4 cup water
1 scant tsp. powdered Agar-Agar
3-4 tbsp. lemon juice
5-6 tbsp. sugar
2 eggs

Prepare as for Orange Cream, Recipe no. 213.

---

* Only from fruits which have not been treated with DDT and
Diphenyl.
** Use only fruit that has not been treated with DDT and Diphenyl.

216. Orange Molds

1-1/4 cups orange juice
1/2 tbsp. Agar-Agar (powdered)*
1 tbsp. sugar
3/4 cup orange juice

Whisk Agar-Agar into 1-1/4 cup orange juice; add sugar. Heat slowly over gentle heat until Agar-Agar is completely dissolved (do not allow to boil). Add the rest of the orange juice. Pour into individual molds previously rinsed out in cold water. Refrigerate until set.

217. Vanilla Sauce

1-1/4 cups milk
1/2 vanilla bean
1 tbsp. sugar
1/2 tsp. cornstarch
1 egg

Prepare as for Vanilla Cream, Recipe no. 207.

218. Almond Milk Sauce

1-3/4 cups milk
2 oz. almonds, peeled, grated
1-1/2 oz. sugar
1 tbsp. cornstarch
2 tbsp. water

Add almonds and sugar to milk and bring to the boil. Mix cornstarch with water, then add to the boiling milk, stirring continuously.

---

* See note for recipe no. 140.

219. Rose Hip Sauce

3 oz. rose hip purée
3/4 cup water or grape juice
3 oz. sugar
Lemon juice (opt.)

Bring purée, water and sugar to the boil. Add a few drops of lemon juice, if desired.

220. Red Grape Sauce

3/4 cup water
Lemon or orange peel
1 stick cinnamon
1 clove
2 to 2-1/2 oz. sugar
3/4 cup red grape juice
1 oz. almonds

Boil the water, peel, cinnamon, clove and sugar together for a few minutes. Strain, add grape juice, heat but do not boil again. Peel almonds, cut into slivers and add to sauce.

221. Fruit Punch

1-1/3 cups water
1 quarter lemon
1/4 stick cinnamon
1 clove
1-1/3 cups apple juice
1-1/3 cups red grape juice
1 tbsp. lemon juice
4 tbsp. sugar
3 tbsp. fruit syrup

Boil water, lemon and spices for 5 min. Strain. Add apple and grape juice, heat again; add lemon juice, sugar and syrup. Serve as hot as possible.

222. Farina Molds

5 oz farina
6 cups milk
2-3 tbsp. sugar
Grated peel of 1 lemon*
1 egg
1-1/2 oz. peeled and grated almonds
1 oz. raisins.

Cook farina as in recipe for Farina Pudding, (Recipe no. 171). Add sugar last of all. Beat egg and add with lemon peel, almonds and raisins. Fill small molds, previously rinsed in cold water. Serve with raspberry syrup.

223. Rice and Lemon Pudding

3-3/4 cups water
Juice of 1 lemon
Chopped lemon peel
5 oz. sugar
5 oz. white pearl rice

Bring water to the boil with lemon juice, peel, and sugar. Add rice, cook for 1/2 hr., cool. Fill mold, previously rinsed in cold water and refrigerate.

---

* Use only fruit not treated with DDT or Diphenyl.

224. Almond Flammeri

4 cups milk
Grated peel of 1 lemon
3-1/2 oz. cornstarch
1 cup milk
3 oz. almonds
3 tbsp. sugar
2 eggs
Raspberry syrup

Bring 4 cups milk and grated lemon peel to the boil. Mix cornstarch with 1 cup milk, add to the boiling milk and lemon. Cook for 5 min. Peel and grate almonds and add with sugar to the hot mixture. Beat the eggs and fold into the cooled mixture. Rinse a mold in cold water and pour pudding into it. Refrigerate, to set. Turn out and serve with raspberry or other fruit syrup.

225. Almond Pudding

2 oz. butter
3-1/2 oz. sugar
3 egg yolks
3-1/2 oz. almonds
6 oz. bread
1 oz. butter
Milk
3 egg whites
1-1/2 oz. raisins
Cinnamon

Beat butter and sugar until creamy, add egg yolks. Peel almonds, roast lightly then grate, add to mixture. Cut thin slices of bread and brown in hot butter; then soak in a little milk and add to the mixture. Beat egg whites to a stiff froth, mix carefully with remaining ingredients. Fold carefully into mixture. Put into a mold and steam over boiling water or in a double boiler for 1 hr. Serve with fruit or Red Grape Sauce, Recipe no. 220.

226. Red Fruit Shape

3 cups blackberry, raspberry or strawberry juice
1-1/4 cups red grape juice or water
2-1/2 oz. farina
1 tbsp. cornstarch

Boil juices together. Stir in farina and cornstarch. Cook for 10 min. Rinse mold in cold water, and fill. Refrigerate to set. Serve with Vanilla Sauce, Recipe no. 217.

227. Baked Lemon Sweet

3 oz. butter
1 cup flour
1-1/2 cups milk
5-1/2 oz. sugar
3 eggs
Grated lemon peel*
2 tbsp. lemon juice

Melt butter, sauté flour in it. Add milk and cook until thick. Take off the flame. Beat sugar, eggs and flavoring. Mix with pudding. Pour into a greased baking dish, steam for 20 min. over boiling water. Bake for a further 20 min. in a moderate oven.

---

* Only from fruits which have not been treated with DDT and Diphenyl.

228. Cottage Cheese Pudding

1-1/2 oz. butter
4 tbsp. flour
1-1/4 cups milk, hot
1 lb. cottage cheese
2 eggs
3 oz. sugar
1-1/2 oz. raisins
Grated lemon peel*

Melt fat, sauté flour in it. Add hot milk and cook for a few minutes, then take off flame. Mix cheese and beaten eggs, then add other ingredients and stir into milk and flour. Grease a deep baking dish and pour mixture into it. Bake in moderate oven for 30-40 min.

229. Apple Fritters

4 tbsp. flour
5 tbsp. water
2 tbsp. apple juice
1 egg white
6 apples (Jonathan)
Vegetable margarine and oil (enough to float the apple slices)
Sugar and cinnamon

Mix flour to a smooth batter with the water and apple juice. Add stiffly beaten egg white. Peel and core the apples and cut slices about 1/2 in. thick. Dip in batter. Fry in deep fat until golden brown. Dip finished fritters in sugar and cinnamon.

---

* Use only unsprayed fruit.

III. Suggested Menus

General Guidelines

Salt: A pinch in cooked vegetables, when permitted.
Fat: No animal fat. Vegetable margarine—butter only rarely (1 oz. per day).
Protein: Use very sparingly. Proteins from whole grains, germ or soy are preferable.

THREE DAY RAW-FOOD DIET

Breakfast: Muesli made with almond purée (with yogurt and raw sugar or honey, when permitted)
                Nuts (all varieties except peanuts)
                Fruit (Rose hip tea in cold weather)

Supper: The same, with the possible use of dried fruit for variety

Lunch: Fruit, nuts (about 1 oz.)
  First day   Raw vegetables: celery, tomatoes, lamb's lettuce
                (The preparation of the dressings is important, see recipes)

Lunch: Second day	Fruit, nuts (about 1 oz.) Raw vegetables: carrots, cucumber, Boston lettuce
Lunch: Third day	Fruit, nuts(about 1 oz.) Raw vegetables: salsify, fennel, endive

SIMPLE MENU FOR ONE WEEK

Breakfast: First day	Muesli prepared with almond milk Whole-grain bread Vegetable margarine or perhaps some butter Nuts Herb tea, raw sugar
Lunch:	Fruit Raw vegetables: cauliflower, Romaine lettuce, corn lettuce Cooked dishes: beans, mashed potatoes Lemon rice pudding
Dinner:	As for breakfast, with the addition of Green spelt soup
Breakfast: Second day	Breakfast for the week is the same as on the first day
Lunch:	Fruit Raw vegetables: kohlrabi, tomatoes, Boston lettuce Cooked dishes: vegetable bouillon (made with onions, leeks, cabbage, potato peel, sorrel), cauliflower, parsley potatoes

Dinner:	As for breakfast, with the addition of Porridge with grapes

Lunch: Third day	Fruit
	Raw vegetables: celeriac, Boston lettuce
	Cooked dishes: Peas in rice ring
	Fruit jello, prepared with Agar-Agar

Dinner:	As above, with addition of Thick potato soup

Lunch: Fourth day	Fruit
	Raw vegetables: Cauliflower, cress
	Cooked dishes: Barley soup, steamed kohlrabi, caraway potatoes

Dinner:	Fruit and nuts
	Vegetable rice
	Plum compote

Lunch: Fifth day	Fruit
	Raw vegetables: Belgian endive or chicory, turnips, cabbage
	Cooked dishes: Romaine lettuce, steamed; toasted rolled oats with soy (instead of eggs)
	Stuffed apple (with grapes and nuts)

Dinner:	As for breakfast, possibly with Soy spread

Lunch: Sixth day	Fruit
	Raw vegetables: Carrots, Brussels sprouts, Boston lettuce
	Cooked dishes: Soy soup, broccoli, steamed; mashed potatoes

Dinner:	As on fifth day

Lunch: Fruit
  Seventh day   Raw vegetables: White radish, Romaine
                 lettuce
                Cooked dishes: Brussels sprouts, steamed;
                 Japanese rice
                Bananas with syrup (no. 191)

Dinner: As above, with addition of cottage cheese
                with chives

EXPANDED MENUS FOR ONE WEEK

Breakfast: (for all seven days)
                Muesli or fruit or fruit juice
                Whole-grain bread
                Butter or vegetable margarine and soy
                 sandwich spread
                Rose hip or herb tea
                Nuts, grated or whole

Dinner: (for all seven days)
                Fruit or fruit salad or 1/2 grapefruit or
                 Muesli
                Add soup; whole-grain bread with cheese;
                 or with tomatoes and oil (grate half a
                 tomato onto the bread and dribble a
                 little olive oil on it in the Spanish
                 style); or baked potatoes with cottage
                 cheese and herbs and salad; or an open-
                 faced sandwich and salad, yogurt, etc.

First day: Fruit, dried fruit
  Lunch   Raw vegetables: Carrots, endive, Boston
                 lettuce
                Vegetable broth with croutons

Salsify with lemon and vegetable margarine
Tomatoes and potatoes

Second day: Fruit, dried fruit
Raw vegetables: Beetroots, cucumbers,
cress
Tomatoes filled with rice
Lemon cream

Third day: Fruit
Raw vegetables: Celeriac, tomatoes,
lamb's lettuce
Farina soup (no. 65)
Chopped kale
Potatoes with caraway

Fourth day: Fruit
Raw vegetables: White radishes, zucchini,
Boston lettuce
Corn bread
Apple cream

Fifth day: Fruit
Raw vegetables: Salsify, spinach, endive
Vegetable soup
Spinach beet stalks with Béchamel sauce
Bouillon potatoes

Sixth day: Fruit
Raw vegetables: Cauliflower, cress, Bos-
ton lettuce
Chervil soup with tomato sauce
Spinach noodles

Seventh day: Fruit
Raw vegetables: Raw tomatoes filled with
celery root salad and potato salad

Steamed Chinese artichokes with lemon juice

Mashed potatoes with tomatoes and herbs

Almond pudding with raspberry syrup

TYPES OF TEA

Diuretic:
  a) Rose hip tea—1 handful of rose hips in 4 cups of water, soak for 12 hours, then allow to simmer for about two hours
  b) Solidago tea—Brew and let steep for 5 minutes
  c) Pansy tea—Brew and let steep for 5 minutes

Relaxant:
  a) Lemon Verbena—Brew and let steep for 5 minutes
  b) Lemon balm tea—Brew and let steep for 5 minutes
  c) Orange blossom tea—brew and let steep for 5 minutes